ACUPUNCTURE FOR PHYSICIANS

ACUPUNCTURE FOR PHYSICIANS

By

TERUO MATSUMOTO, M.D., Ph.D., F.A.C.S.

Professor of Surgery, Director, Division of Surgical Research,
Critical Care Laboratory, and Shock and Trauma Unit,
Hahnemann Medical College and Hospital, Philadelphia
Senior Attending Surgeon
Philadelphia General Hospital, Philadelphia
Consultant
Valley Forge U. S. Army Hospital
Valley Forge, Pennsylvania

CHARLES C THOMAS • PUBLISHER
Springfield • Illinois • U. S. A.

Published and Distributed Throughout the World by

CHARLES C THOMAS • PUBLISHER

BANNERSTONE HOUSE

301-327 East Lawrence Avenue, Springfield, Illinois, U.S.A.

ISBN 0-398-02958-X

Library of Congress Catalog Card Number: 75-10186

With THOMAS BOOKS *careful attention is given to all details of manufacturing and design. It is the Publisher's desire to present books that are satisfactory as to their physical qualities and artistic possibilities and appropriate for their particular use.* THOMAS BOOKS *will be true to those laws of quality that assure a good name and good will.*

Printed in the United States of America

HH-11

Library of Congress Cataloging in Publication Data

Matsumoto, Teruo.

Acupuncture for physicians.

1. Acupuncture. I. Title. [DNLM: 1. Acupuncture.
WB369 M434a 1973]

RM184.M38 615'.892 73-10186

ISBN 0-398-02958-X

FOREWORD

Recent reports from the Peoples Republic of China on the value of acupuncture, as well as the lack of information on its scientific foundation, have given the public and the medical profession the impression that acupuncture is rather empirical and that one may, not unjustly, treat it with skepticism. Accordingly, I have reviewed the abundant original descriptions of acupuncture written in foreign languages and undertaken a trip to Japan, where many patients who have received acupuncture treatment have experienced relief from the pain of some illnesses.

To understand acupuncture one begins by learning about meridian points, certain points on the body surface that correspond specifically to the particular diseased organ. These points have been discovered by actual experience of more than 3,000 years with the use of acupuncture needles. The needles used in acupuncture come in varying sizes, some as thin as 0.14 mm in diameter. The procedure is considered simple, painless, and generally, no appreciable risk is involved. According to modern medical concepts, many of the meridian points correspond to areas where vessels and nerves are located relatively superficially, such as in areas between muscle and bone, or between bone and joint. In addition, some of these points are considered "electropermeable points," which are electrically less resistant than other areas.[1] "Head and McKenzie's sensory zone," which radiates visceral pain to certain parts of the skin by sending impulses via the autonomic nerve in the viscera and a sympathetic fiber,[2] shows some relationship to the meridian point.

Explanation of the pathophysiological basis of acupuncture using the old Chinese *five elements theory*[3] should be abandoned in favor of the electrophysiologic concept, Reverse Head-McKenzie theory, and the gate control system theory proposed by Melzack and Wall.[4] A gate control system modulates sensory input from the skin before it evokes pain, perception, and response. The findings of groups of vagus nerve endings in the pinna of the ear through the technique of myelin sheath staining[5] may help to explain the relationships that can exist between two anatomically separated areas.

The introduction of electrical current for the purpose of local or regional anesthesia, as practiced in China, is an entirely new concept of anesthesia. However, it should be remembered that the development became possible because of the existence of traditional Chinese medicine-acupuncture. An article on "Acupuncture Anesthesia" which appeared recently in *The Jour-*

nal[5] describes the application of direct current as a type of irritation. According to existing medical knowledge, the effect of stimulation with electric current (direct current) is to create sudden changes in electric polarization,[6] in addition to the *injury current* created by the piercing of needles. The application of electrical current to acupuncture needles placed in the meridian points increases the efficacy of acupuncture in controlling pain. This well-known effect is now being practiced at Japanese medical schools.

Modern medicine as developed in the western hemisphere and now practiced throughout the world appears to be highly effective in the cure of disease. However, there are still certain conditions and diseases for which modern medicine is not indicated or even effective. At present, incurable diseases and discomfort accompanying various illnesses still exist. Chronic pain frequently becomes a problem for the patients themselves, their family, and even the nation.

Acupuncture may yet prove valuable in our modern practice as a method of easing pain and producing a type of anesthesia. Since we do not have an answer for the mechanism of acupuncture, further evaluation of acupuncture must be undertaken on a scientific basis. Neurophysiologic evaluation, including skin resistance, and anatomic distribution of autonomic nerve fibers of meridian or acupuncture points and study of their ultrastructure must be undertaken in relation to acupuncture both with or without electric current. The objective analysis of the efficacy of acupuncture by well-controlled, double-blind studies with reasonable statistical analysis should be made by a multidisciplinary approach.

Acupuncture at present is still experimental in this country. To evaluate acupuncture, The National Institute of Health organized an *ad hoc* committee and appointed as its chairman John J. Bonica, M.D. who is professor and chairman of the Department of Anesthesiology, Washington University. Under his direction, the first acupuncture conference was held at NIH from the 28th of February to the 1st of March.[7] It was the conclusion of the conference that the efficacy of acupuncture is not known at this time. It was further concluded that a careful and controlled study should be conducted at the appropriate medical schools.

The public's knowledge concerning acupuncture is extremely limited and only its advantages have been emphasized. Even though it has been well documented that a thoracotomy was successfully performed under acupuncture anesthesia, it is not known what *types* of pre-anesthesia preparations *were* made (intensive pulmonary physical-therapy, artificial pneumothorax training of abdominal breathing, etc.). In addition, it is essential to know the blood gas during anesthesia. One wonders if this procedure is still in use and if so, under what indications.

It will become a national medical disaster if patients receive acupuncture for pain without first having a proper workup, since pain is often the first alarm of various illnesses. One may, in fact, lose a golden period of time during which modern medical technology could have eradicated the disease. A prime example of this is cancer. My own personal experience was such that a patient, seen by an acupuncturist elsewhere, requested me to continue acupuncture in order to reduce pain at the right upper quadrant of the abdomen which later proved to be chololithiasis. In addition, patients are often reluctant to return to their approved physician since the physician was unhappy to know of the patient's desire to receive acupuncture treatment. Yet, the physician was unable to explain how or why acupuncture works.

Therefore, it is the intention of this author to provide adequate clinical knowledge of acupuncture, as practiced in the orient, in order that the physicians may communicate the practical aspects of acupuncture to their confused patients. In addition to providing physicians with the appropriate knowledge of acupuncture in order that they may explain acupuncture to their patients, this book is also prepared to prevent the patient from seeking acupuncture prematurely. It is not the objective of this book to encourage the blind practice of acupuncture.

Although the basis of this book is my personal clinical experiences, indications of acupuncture for various diseases are merely based on the oriental literature except for the part concerning muscular-skeletal pain. Clinical anesthesia is based on the literature received from The Republic of China and Japan; however, experimental studies are based on my own experiences.

Teruo Matsumoto

ACKNOWLEDGMENTS

I duly acknowledge the following list of articles which appear in this book and extend my appreciation to the publishers for their cooperation in allowing me to include this material as part of the book:

Acupuncture and U. S. medicine, *Jama, 220*:1010, May, 1972.

Acupuncture electric phenomenon of the skin and postvagotomy gastrointestinal atony, *Am J Surg, 125*:176, February 1973.

Acupunctures; *Am Surg,* and *Int Surg,* to be published.

I would also like to acknowledge the work of Mr. Nolan Jones, research instructor in the Department of Surgery, Mr. Ronald Deitrick and Miss Jeanette Kienle, M.T. Numerous valuable informations were provided by Dr. M. Miyata, Jiyosei Dental College, Japan.

This work was supported in part by the Samuel S. Fels Foundation, through the generosity of Mr. Charles Conway and Wharton Shober, President, Hahnemann Medical College and Hospital.

T. M.

CONTENTS

Page

Foreword . . . . *v*

Acknowledgments . . . . *ix*

Chapter

1. INTRODUCTION AND BASIC KNOWLEDGE OF ACUPUNCTURE 3
2. CLINICAL PRACTICE OF ACUPUNCTURE 23
3. ACUPUNCTURE ANESTHESIA 89
4. ACUPUNCTURE RESEARCH 97
5. PROPOSED RESEARCH 151
6. ADDITIONAL STUDIES 171

Appendices

I Acupuncture Points (English Terms) 196

II Acupuncture Points (Oriental Terms) 198

Index 200

ACUPUNCTURE FOR PHYSICIANS

CHAPTER 1

INTRODUCTION AND BASIC KNOWLEDGE OF ACUPUNCTURE

HISTORICAL REVIEW

According to most reports acupuncture seems to have been developed in the northern-most area of the mainline of China around 300 B.C.

People in this area were primarily nomads, moving from one area to another in an attempt to avoid cold weather. Because of the climatic factor it was not desirable for them to remove their clothing for medical treatment. This necessitated the development of a method of treatment that stimulated an exposed area such as the head and extremities. During these early times, it was noted that certain points of the body responded more noticeably to stimulation than other points and that frequently there was a direct correlation between the points responsive and a particular ailment. These certain points were subsequently named *Meridian Points*.[8] At a later time, when metal was introduced to the culture, needles were used as an irritant at meridian points, and it was thought that pain from a specific ailment was diverted in a linear fashion through the meridian points to the surface of the body. Thus, the concept of *Meridian Line* was developed.[8]

The earliest book describing acupuncture was written in 50 B.C. It described the clinical applications of acupuncture with anatomical and physiological references based principally on the concept of the meridian lines of the body.[9]

In 1911, Sonbun, who had trained in a modern western culture, formed the Republic of China. Under his rule, old Chinese medicine, including acupuncture which had developed from tradition and experience, was not able to survive except in outlying areas of China.

However, when Mao-Tse-Tung, in 1949, formed the People's Republic of China, he tried to re-popularize the old methods of Chinese medicine which had been so helpful to him. In the 1930's when he and his followers were retreating to the North he was forced to depend mainly on these traditional methods for medical treatment.

In 1955, Shyuken, a follower of Mao-Tse-Tung, stated his belief that acupuncture was effective in the management of the ill. He wanted to study the old Chinese way of medicine more systemically, comparing it to western medicine, which he believed to be too analytical.[10] Thus, a new medical movement began uniting western and Chinese medical practices.

MERIDIAN POINTS

Stimulation therapy by local heat, massage, and pressure has been known since ancient times. The observations and analysis by Chinese physicians over long periods of time of the effects on signs and symptoms, following irritation of varying degrees at some certain points on the body surface, made it possible to relate the most effective points on the body to specific conditions. These were named meridian points.[8]

According to the ancient Chinese clinical concepts, the meridian points served as *peeping holes* into the body and *passing holes* for energy. The total number of meridian points was believed to be 365.[11] Each was named by its effect, anatomical location, appearance, and relation to the meridian line. These meridian points were selected initially according to measurements based on the patient's own unique anatomical standard (using the length between certain anatomical points, for example, between nipples) (Fig. 1). The exact location of a meridian point is then selected by the examiner who feels with his finger tips the areas chosen by the initial measurement and watches the patient's response.

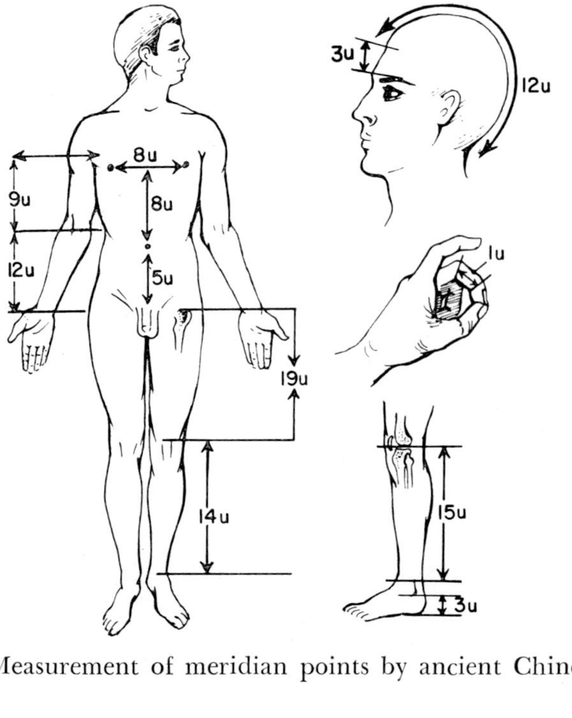

Figure 1: Measurement of meridian points by ancient Chinese method.

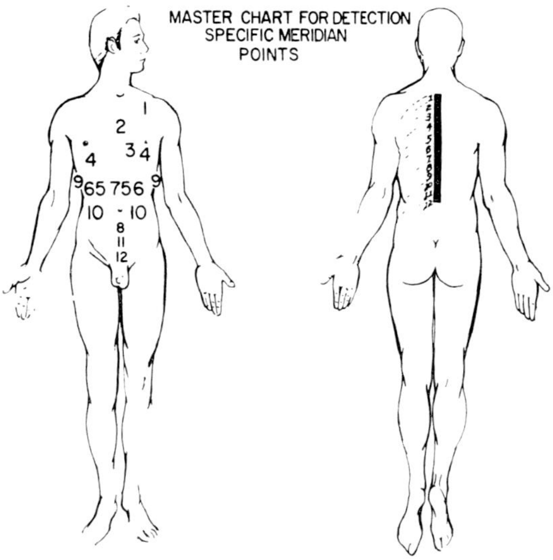

Figure 2: Tenderness at numbered areas in this figure corresponds to the associated disease organ and the specific meridian points in Table I.

According to modern medical concepts, some of these points will be best elucidated by use of a neurometer to electrically define the less resistive areas.[12] In addition, some are thought to be relating points in which the autonomic nerve system is stimulated by a specific visceral disorder. Anatomically, some of the meridian points seem to correspond to an area where a nerve appears to surface from a muscle or an area where vessels and nerves are located relatively superficially, such as in areas between a muscle and a bone, a bone and a joint, etc.[12] These areas are generally composed of connective tissue. Details will be discussed in the latter portion of the book.

Each of the twelve points in the front and back of the body represents the related organ. When one feels the specific point which is sensitive, painful

Table I
Major Meridian Lines Correspond to the Points in Figure 3

Number in Fig. 2	Name of Meridian Line	Figure 3 Letter
1	Pulmonary	a
2	Colonic	f
3	Gastric	h, i
4	Splenic	k
5	Cardiac	b
6	Intestinal	d
7	Urinary Bladder	m, n
8	Renal	o
9	Vascular	c
10	Endocrine	e
11	Biliary	g, l
12	Hepatic	j

or hard by palpation, the point is considered to be abnormal (Fig. 2). Each number of Figure 2 corresponds to the meridian line in Figure 3 and to the meridian points as shown in Table I, as well as the associated diseased organ.[13-17] The examination of this point in Figure 3, therefore, is somewhat useful for diagnosis of disorders and determination of the specific points on the meridian line to be treated by acupuncture. The major meridian lines and points are shown in Figure 3, A-P, which follows. The points described have been evaluated by electric resistance (Fig. 4), myography, and pulse wave. It is reported that some of these points certainly represent a disorder of each internal organ.[12,13]

ELECTRICAL ACUPUNCTURE

"Anesthesia for major surgery" was the subtitle of an article which was published in *Infectious Diseases* on July 3, 1971.[18] The article goes on to

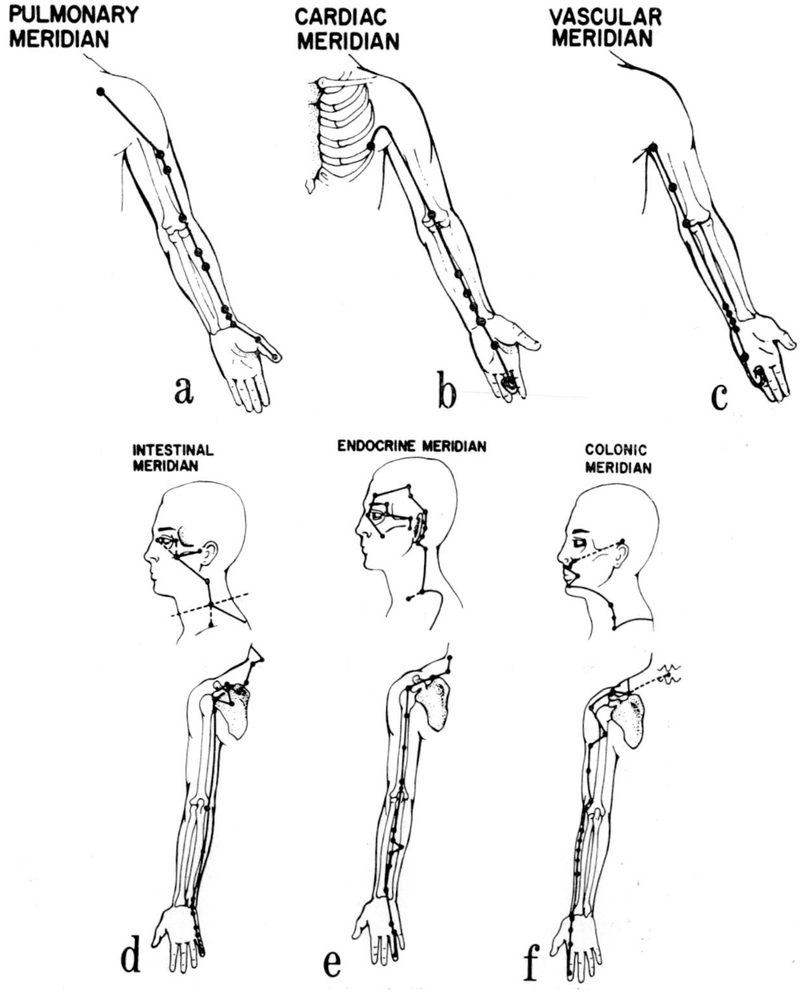

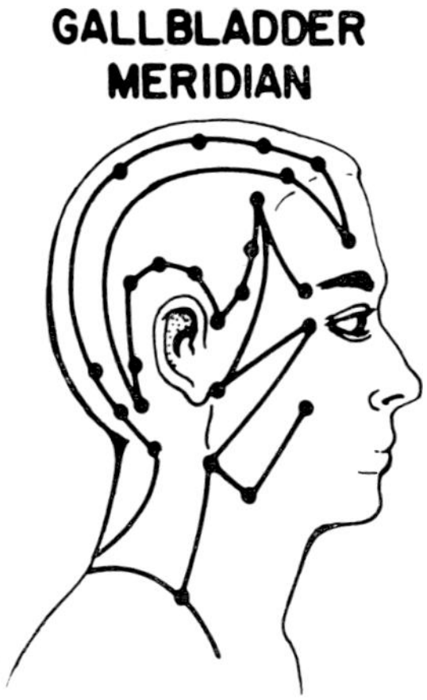

g

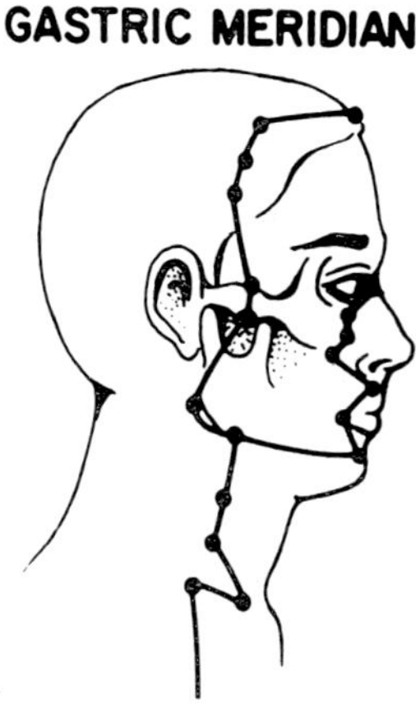

h

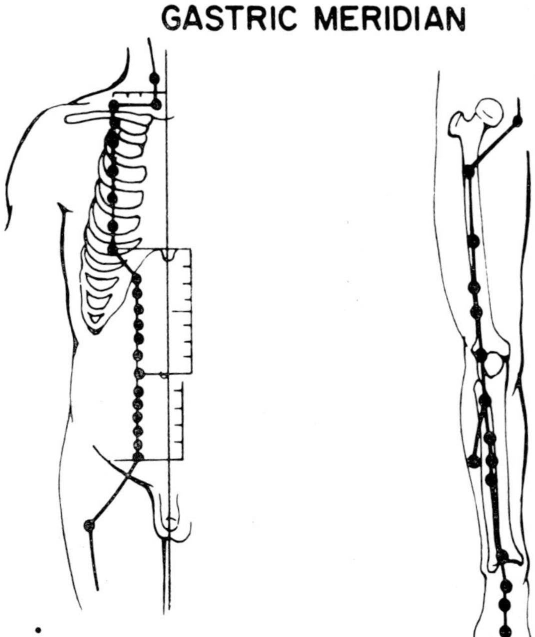

i

state "in patients being prepared for abdominal surgery, two needles were placed in the abdomen and two in the legs. In the patients requiring thyroid surgery, two needles were placed in the neck and one in each wrist. Then, needles were hooked to a single electrical device and the current was turned on. The thyroid patient had not only these four implanted electrodes but also two on the surface taped to the chest. A current of 5 volts and 200 microamperes was applied for 20 minutes.

In a recent issue of the *Journal of the American Medical Association*

HEPATIC MERIDIAN

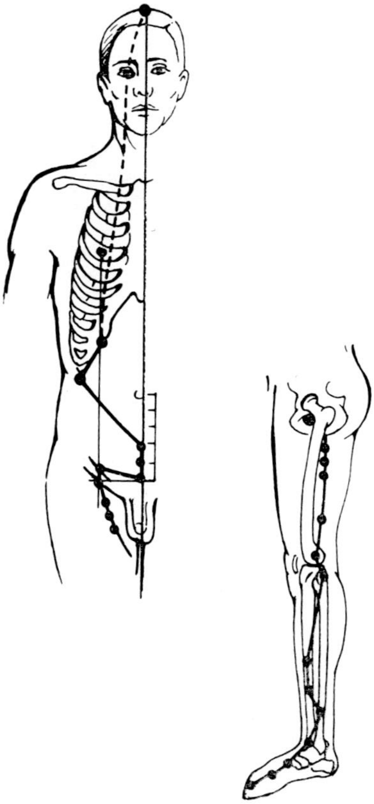

j

SPLENIC MERIDIAN

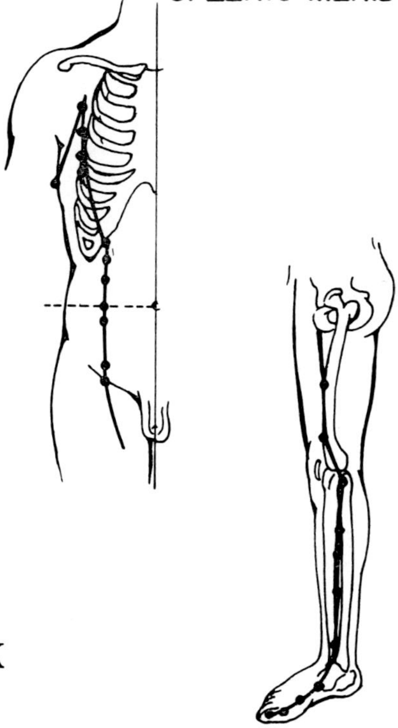

k

BILIARY MERIDIAN

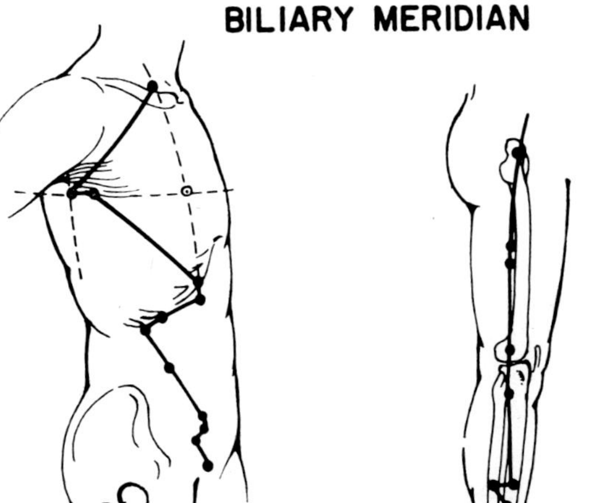

l

URINARY BLADDER MERIDIAN

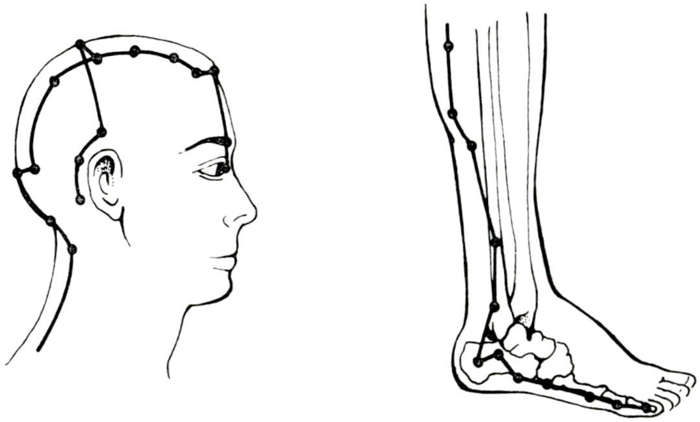

m

BLADDER MERIDIAN

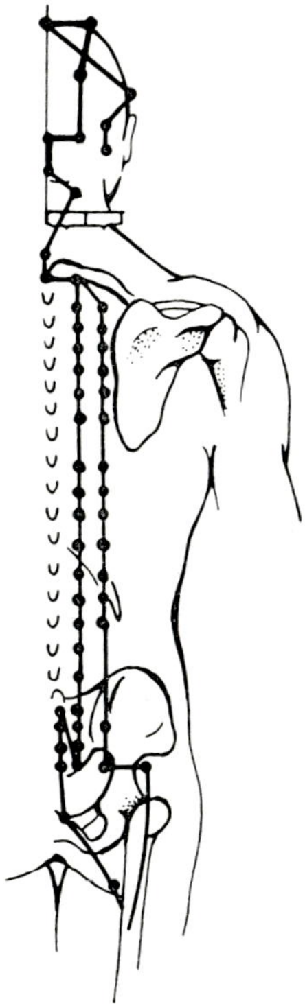

n

RENAL MERIDIAN

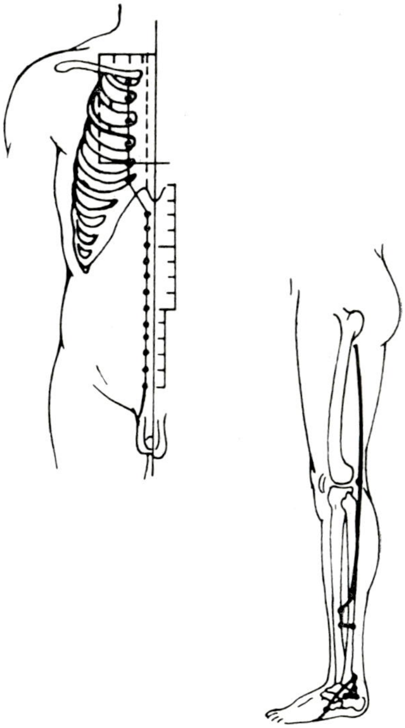

o

a similar report was published.[19] The key to the anesthesia in this situation must be the application of acupuncture needles and constant stimulation —electric stimulation in these cases. Effect of stimulation by electric energy is many times stronger than that of mechanical energy. DC current is the

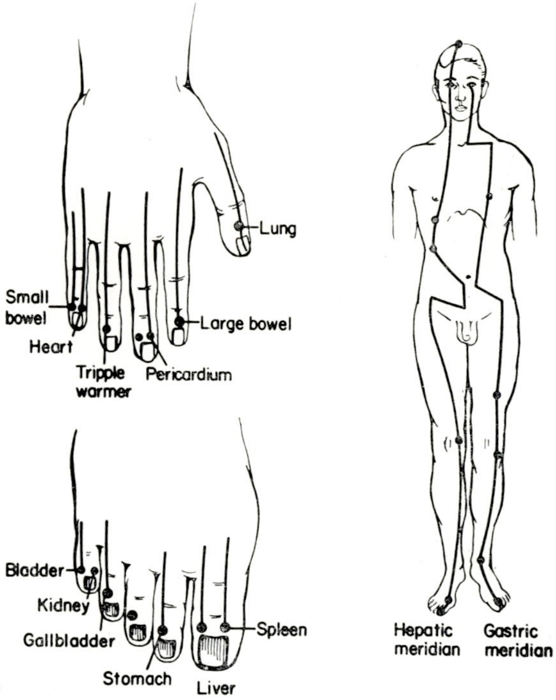

p

Figure 3:

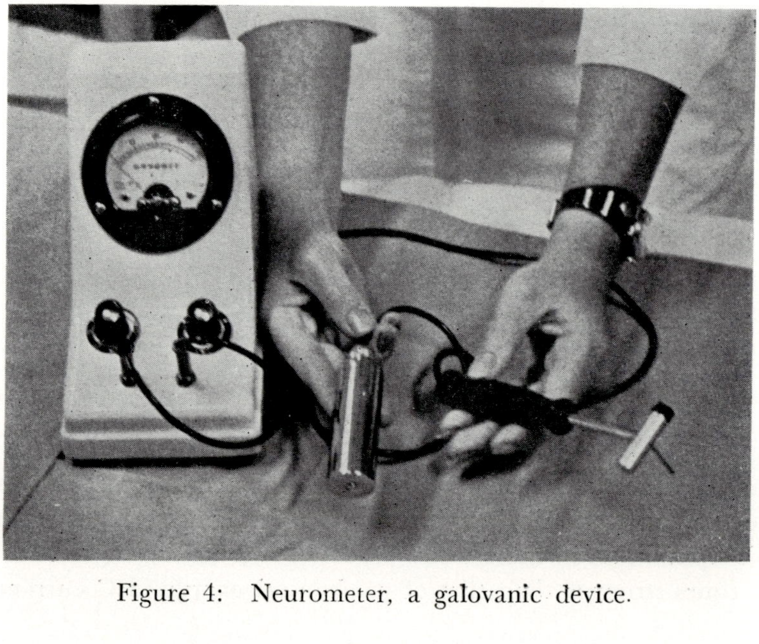

Figure 4: Neurometer, a galovanic device.

most effective electrical energy for this use. It is known that DC current is not mandatory. Destruction of cells by the placing of needles causes an injury current and the additional DC current supplied causes sudden changes in electrical polarization. This may be the reason for the rapid anti-pain effect following application of electrical acupuncture. When voltage is increased, the sensory nerve is also anesthetized. Ten to fifteen volts, however, may not be effective on the sensory nerve, although reportedly the degree of tension on the sympathetic nerve has a great influence on this sensory factor.[12]

Application of electric current with acupuncture needles placed on the meridian points increases the efficacy of acupuncture to control pain. This has been well known and practiced at pain clinics at Osaka Medical College in Japan.[12]

Use of electric current as a method of general anesthesia had been tried without success in western medicine.[20-38]

In China, where the best anesthesia equipment may not always be available and well trained anesthetists may be scarce, local and regional anesthesia which can be administered with minimum knowledge and skill may be widely used out of necessity. These situations may have contributed more to the development of a new mode of anesthesia. Introduction of electrical current for the purpose of local or regional anesthesia as practiced in China is thus an entirely new mode. However, it should be remembered that this development became possible because of the existence of the traditional Chinese medicine–acupuncture. Also the use of electric

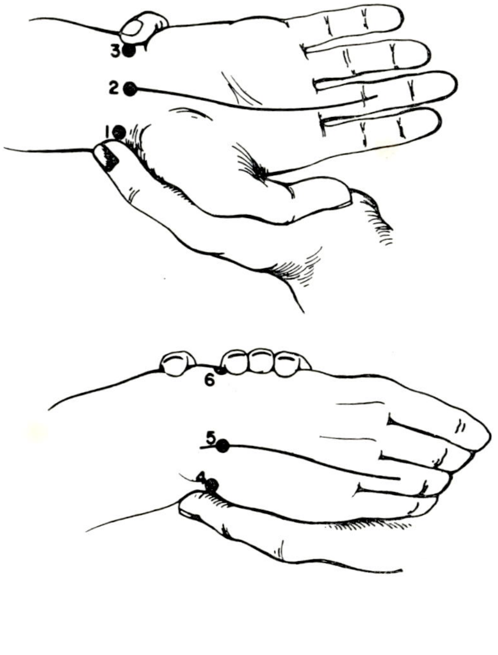

Figure 5: Representative measurement points (wrist).

current (as an alternative method of stimulation) has been used for the practice of acupuncture and is not a new concept.

General Ryodoraku Regulation Therapy

In oriental medicine there are two modes of treatment. These are general and local.

General or essential treatment is primarily to balance positive and negative in the meridian line. Ryodoraku literally means the line where electric permiability is increased. According to the Ryodoraku theory, abnormal Ryodoraku indicates increased or decreased amount of electricity on the meridian. This will be measured by simply adding the measured electric units on the specific points on the meridian and dividing the units by the number of the specific points.

According to experiences, it is possible to measure only a representative point instead of the above. Thus, in order to determine abnormality of the specific meridian line, one representative point at each meridian line has been selected (Figs. 5 and 6). Measuring the electric unit at these representative points, the Ryodoraku chart can be completed and the value may be evaluated by the standard.

PAIN AND ACTING POINTS OF PAIN MANAGEMENT

Excluding pain caused by cerebral pathology, there are certain mechanisms of pain which are recognized.[38] These are causal factors (stimuli), such as the inflammation or trauma, the receptor, the peripheral nervous system, and the brain.

1. Removal of Causal Factor:

   This is the basic principle of modern medicine. However, such disease causing pain may not be cured instantaneously, and management of pain must depend on other means until the disease is cured.

2. Control of Chemical Reaction on Receptor and Reduction of Sensitivity of Receptor:

   Intensive studies have been done concerning the stimulation causing

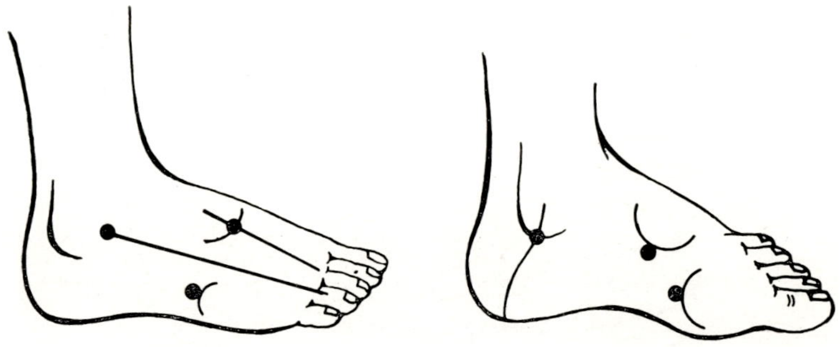

Figure 6: Representative measure points (foot).

pain. A recent study indicated that essential for pain are intrinsic chemical substances (polypeptides) such as histamine, serotonin, bradikinin, K H^+, and acetylcholine which stimulate the receptor. Therefore, an antagonistic drug for these chemicals may be effective for pain control. Aspirin is thought to be antagonistic for many of these chemicals.

Topical hypothermia and local anesthetics are effective for surface pain in order to reduce sensitivity of the receptor.

3. Interruption of the Pathway of Stimulation: Nerve Block represents this Mechanism.
4. Changing the Pattern with Time and Frequency of Stimulation from Peripheral Nerve to Central Nervous System:
   Stimulation therapy is representative of this mechanism. Acupuncture certainly belongs in the category of stimulation therapy. Also, dorsal column stimulation can be included here.
5. Interruption of the Pathway of Stimulation in Spinal Cord and Brain: Neurosurgical intervention such as rhizotomy, chordotomy and tractotomy. Thalamotomy and recently cingulotomy are used alone or in conjunction with the above methods and account for this category.
6. Sedative Control of Pain:
   The majority of sedatives and tranquilizers probably act on the Limbic Lobe of the brain. Some of the sedatives may act on the

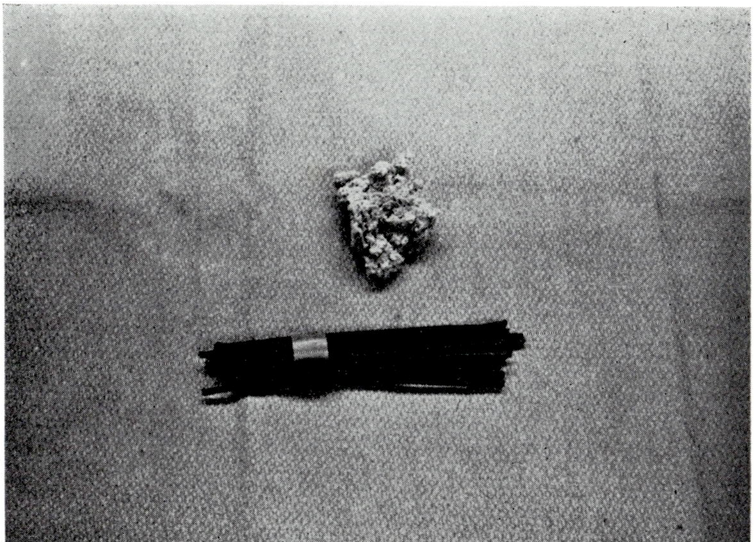

Figure 7: Moxa and incense sticks.

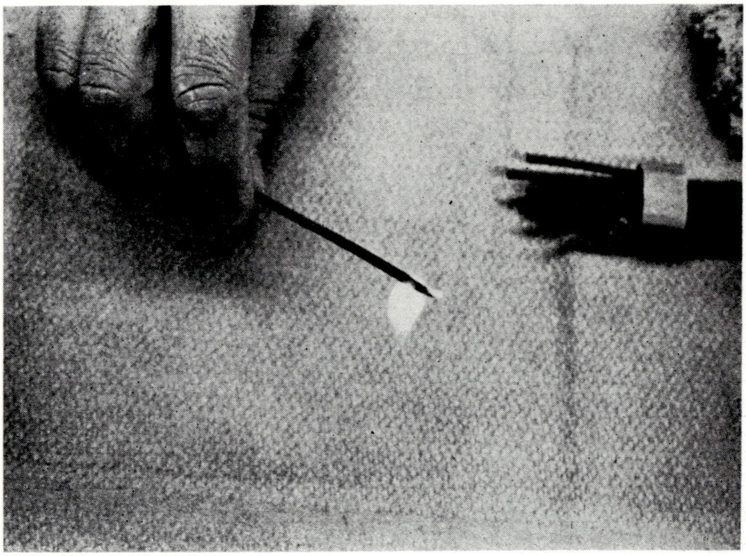

Figure 8: An incense stick is being lit.

passage of pain sensation in the brain stem but they control recognition of pain in general at higher cerebral levels.

ACUPUNCTURE AND STIMULATION THERAPY

Acupuncture is one mode of stimulation therapy and the mechanism is due to changing the pattern of passage of stimulation from peripheral nerves to the central nervous system.

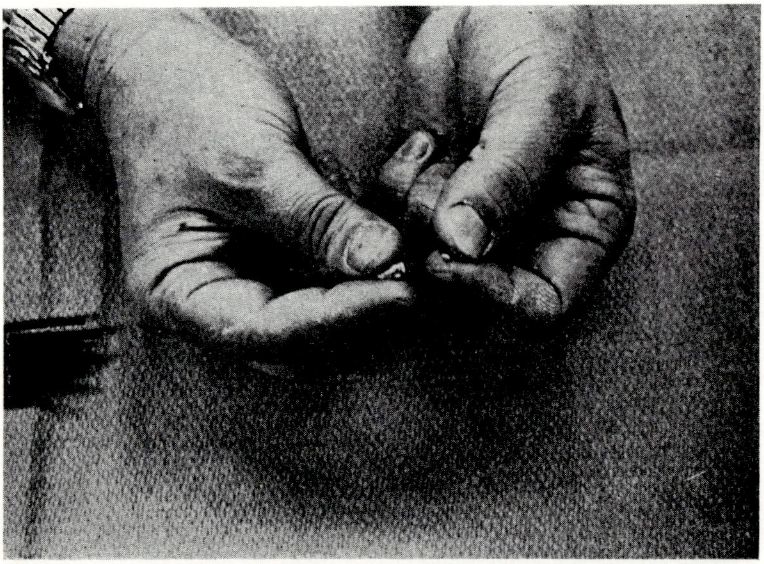

Figure 9: Moxa is now being divided.

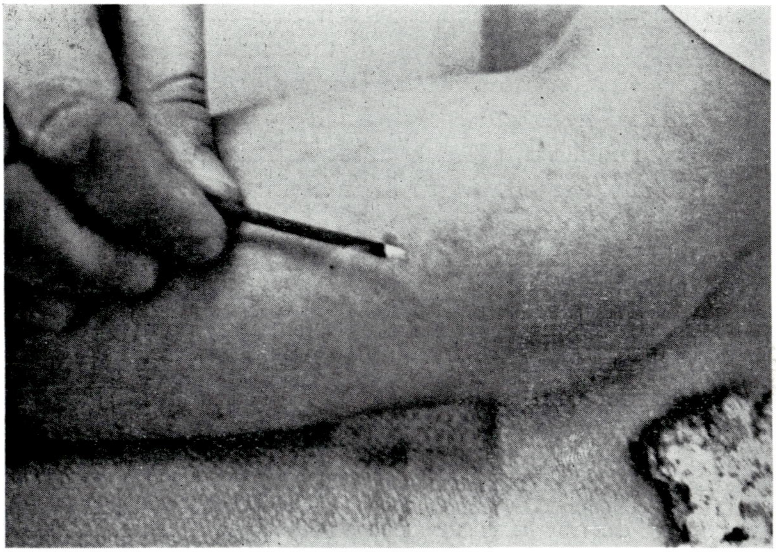

Figure 10: Moxa is placed on the meridian point and lit with the incense stick.

Stimulation therapy such as hot soaks and management of certain pain problems with physical therapy has existed and been established in human society. Oriental medicine has accumulated experiences, analyzed the quality of stimulation and organized these to a medical system.

In the beginning, meridian points which were effective for certain ailments were organized and special names were given to each for improving

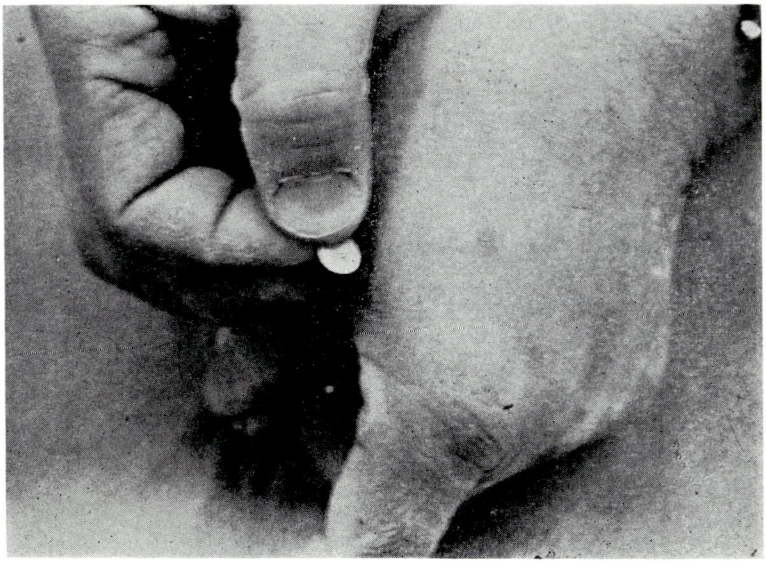

Figure 11: A metalic ball is placed at the center of small band-aid.

their understanding. Then, the meridian line concept was hypothesized in order to explain the effectiveness of the meridian points. Since these meridian points were selected by the observation of the effect of stimulation on the special signs and symptoms, it is reasonable to believe these points could be used advantageously in modern medicine. However, pathophysiologic explanation of the meridian points have not been adequate and a majority are not explainable by modern medical knowledge.

Another mode of stimulation on the meridian points is moxibustion (Figs. 7-10). Recently a small metalic ball has been used to produce a mild yet constant stimulation on the specific meridian points (Figs. 11, 12). However, these metalic balls occasionally cause superficial but distinct compression necrosis on the skin if they are in place for a long period of time.

BASIC THEORIES OF THE PATHOPHYSIOLOGY OF ACUPUNCTURE

Presently, we do not have an understanding of the mechanism of acupuncture. Some of the theories are as follows:

Meridian Line Theory

"Fever, headache, shoulder ache, cough, heart burn, palpitation, sleeplessness, numbness, etc. are well known symptoms to the medical practitioner. In western medicine, a physician diagnoses a person who has a group of such signs and symptoms as having a specific ailment, such as pneumonia or arteriosclerotic heart disease, and then begins treatment. In contrast,

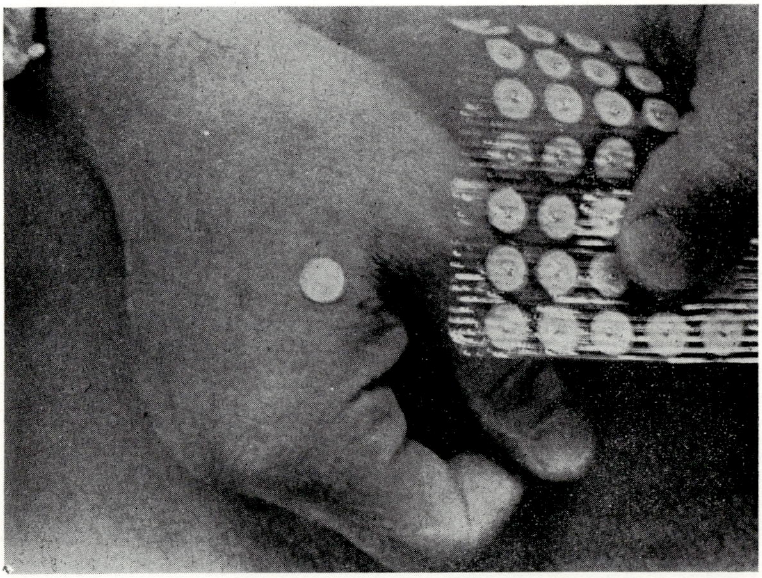

Figure 12: A metalic ball is now attached to a meridian point.

the old Chinese medicine treated patients by a symptoms complex and a pulse diagnosis has been used (Fig. 13).

The basis of this system of oriental medicine was the *six solid and six hollow organs* theory. According to this belief, the following twelve organs control the body: liver, heart, spleen, lung, kidney, and major blood vessels which are solid organs and gallbladder, small bowel, stomach, bladder, large bowel, and endocrine system which are hollow organs. This theory combined the more primitive Chinese concepts of *five elements* and *positive and negative* forces.[39-42]

The five elements theory explained every existing natural and human phenomenom in terms of the five basic elements: wood, heat, soil, metal, and liquid. According to this theory, organs and all pathological findings may be classified under one of the five elements. Thus, the basic five elements in the human are the liver as wood, heart as heat, spleen as soil, lung as metal, and kidney as liquid. Later, five associate organs were named

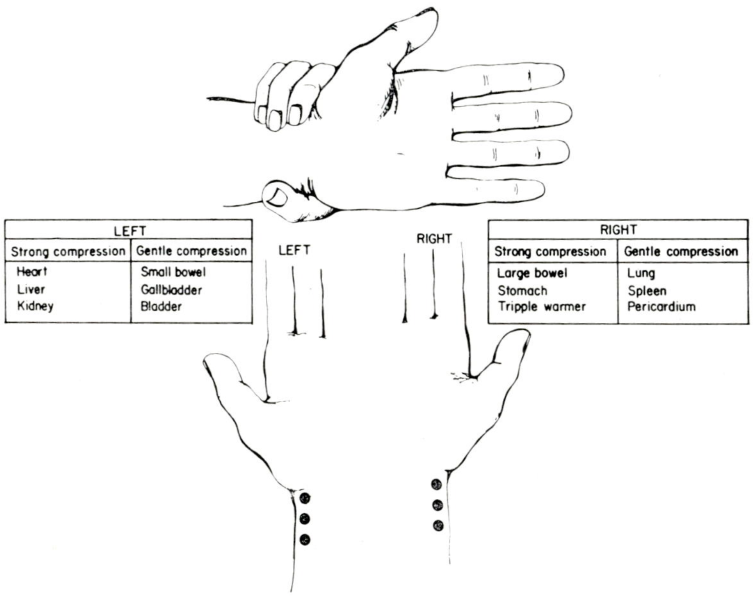

Figure 13: Pulse Diagnosis: Place tip of middle finger over radial styloid processus and obtain the pulse (Kuan). Then, place index and ring finger tips both sides of the middle finger (Tsun and chih respectively). Now compress the riadial artery firmly, (sinking pulse) and gently (floating pulse).

Floating pulse evaluates positive or negative phase of 6 positive organs and sinking pulse measures the same of the 6 negative organs. For example, if the pulse is weak when compress Tsun very gently, the pulse diagnosis indicates negative cardiac line. This method is essential to know the positive or negative phase of meridian line, and it takes 30 years to learn *how to master pulse diagnosis* according to oriental medicine.

as important organs in order to maintain human life. These are the biliary system which corresponds to the liver, small intestine (heart), stomach (spleen), colon (lung) and bladder (kidney). These ten organs were called *5 solid and 5 hollow organs.* Even later two other organs, great vessels and endocrine organs, were added to the above, and the concept of *6 solid and 6 hollow organs* was thus finalized.[43]

What is the relationship between these twelve organs and the meridian point? Why do symptoms reportedly subside or disease remit when acupuncture is applied at certain meridian points? In oriental medicine, a special flow system for energy is thought to exist. This system is felt to provide vital energy to each organ via the meridian line. The meridian lines run longitudinally in the human body, and each meridian line has a name associated with the organ controlling it. Thus these meridian lines are (1) pulmonary, (2) colonic, (3) gastric, (4) splenic, (5) cardiac, (6) small intestine, (7) vesicular, (8) renal, (9) greater vascular, (10) endocrine, (11) biliary, and (12) hepatic (Table II). The correspondence to the six solid and six hollow organs theory is clear and so there are twelve meridian lines in the body (Table II). According to the old Chinese medical philosophy, as long as energy is running through these twelve meridians, the patient is healthy. Meridian points are located on a meridian line (Fig. 3). Needling certain points on a meridian line has a positive effect on the corresponding disease because this balances the energy flow.[10] Intensive study of acupuncture has revealed that it is certainly difficult to accept these concepts as to pathophysiology of a particular disease.

"Rapid needle therapy"[44] by the People's Republic of China Air Force Hospital at Shanyan, was published in November, 1969. Its first edition was printed as 500,000 copies. This indicated to the observer the re-recognition of acupuncture and the popularization of this practice. It is noteworthy to mention that while meridian points were the major subject of this book, no description was noted concerning meridian lines. This seems to indicate the rejection of a meridian line theory based on energy flow and five elements theory in modern Chinese acupuncture.

A report from Korea in 1963 which explained meridian lines by existence

TABLE II

Position	Back (Positive)-Yars	Front (Negative)-Yin	Five Elements
	Back of Hand	*Palm*	
Radial	Colonic-L. I.	Pulmonary (Lung)	Metal
Middle	Endocrine-T. W.	Vascular (Pericardium)	———
Ulnar	Intestinal-S. I.	Cardiac (Heart)	Heat
	Back of Foot	*Sole*	
Tibial	Gastric Stomach	Splenic (Spleen)	Soil
Middle	Biliary Gall Bladder	Hepatic (Liver)	Tree
Fibular	Bladder	Renal (Kidney)	Liquid

Meridian Line and Five Elements

of Bon Han fluid and Bon Han granules by histologic study and use of isotopes has not yet been confirmed by scientists in Japan or China.[12,45] Presently, there is no proven histologic relationship between meridian points and meridian lines. This, of course, is not reason enough to deny completely the existence of the meridian lines. Recent Chinese observation of groupings of vagal nerve endings in the pinna of the ear may reopen a door to re-entry of the concept of meridian lines.

Stress Theory (Hans Selye)

Acupuncture may become a stressor to pituitary-adrenocortical system.[46]

Reilly Phenomenon

Reilly believes the autonomic nervous system is the first stage of an activation and is followed by a reaction of the adrenal glands, while Selye's theory considers that the adrenocortical system function precedes the autonomic nervous system.[46]

Head-McKenzie Zone

The discovery of a *Head-McKenzie sensory zone* which radiates visceral pain to certain parts of the skin[46] (cardiac ischemia with radiation of pain to the left arm) is familiar to us and shows some relationships to the meridian line and point.

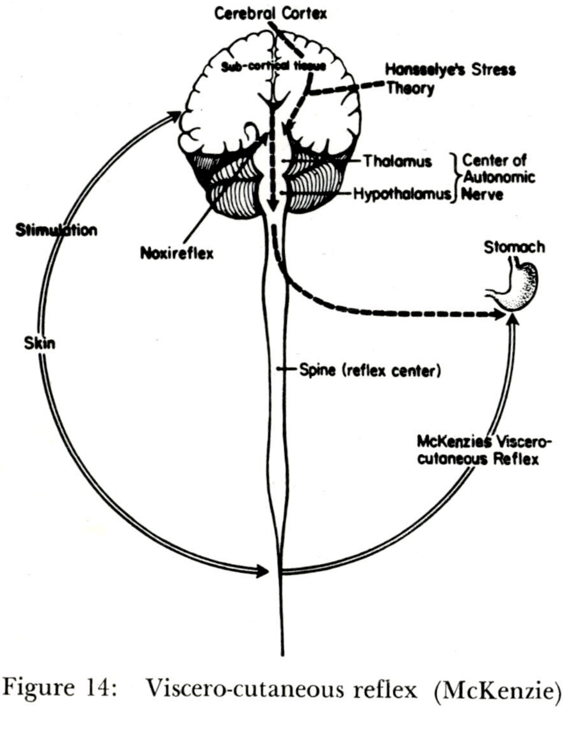

Figure 14: Viscero-cutaneous reflex (McKenzie).

Hiyodo measured electric potential on the skin in patients and found that a special pattern of electropermeable points formed a specific line corresponding to various diseases. His study revealed that the meridian line is actually existent but is nothing more than an electro-permissive phenomena.[12] Since no such pattern existed in healthy people and the presence of the electropermeable line was related to the disease process, he felt the mechanism was attributed to viscero-cutaneous autonomic nerve reflex.[12] Thus, impulses from the viscera reached the spinal cord and the stimulus was projected to the skin through the sympathetic nervous system (Figs. 14, 15).

The fact that (1) electropotential of the skin supplied by the sympathetic nerve system increases and the electro-permeable line disappears with sympathetic block, and (2) stimulation of sympathetic nervous system increases the electro-permeable line may be aids in explaining the above theory. Thus in essence, the meridian line is a functional route by which the sympathetic nerve system reveals stimulation by a visceral disorder and so pathological conditions allow stimulation from diseased organs to form hypersensitive points on the body surface. These particular points are called *paraviose*.[12] In these situations exudate accumulates in paraviose and swelling of mitocondria is seen.

Such local circulation disturbances eventually cause abnormal excitation of the autonomic nervous system.[12] The area of the paraviose is unusually stimulated and electrically depolarized compared to an area of normal stimulation. Since a depolarized condition reduces dermal electrical resistance, these points become electrically permeable points. Thus, the use of a neurometer and detection of conduction points may help to prove the existences of abnormal points, which may be considered as meridian points.

Finally, appropriate stimulation by acupuncture on these reactive electropermissible points sends impulses centrally via a sympathetic afferent fiber and the autonomic nerve in the viscera is regulated by the reverse of the McKenzie theory (Figs. 14, 15).

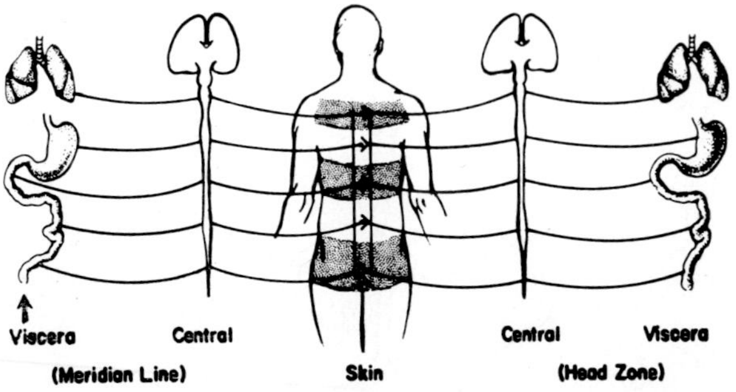

Figure 15: Viscero-cutaneous reflex, Meridian line versus head zone.

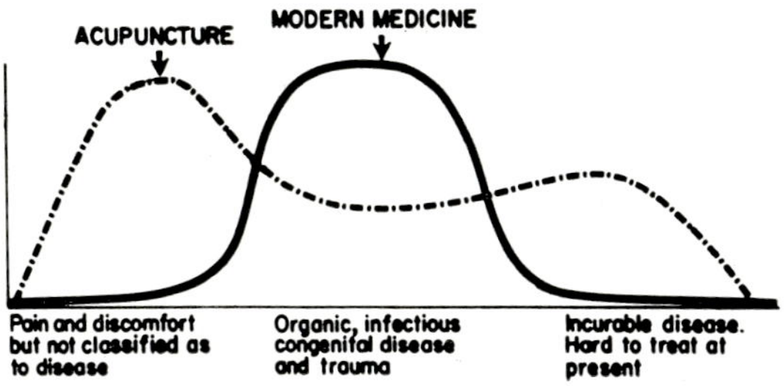

Figure 16: Proven efficacy of modern medicine versus possible efficacy of acupuncture.

Accordingly, an electric potential applied to the reactive electro-permissible points reduces this flow and the symptoms subside.

Gate Control Theory

Impulse to the large alpha and beta fiber initiated by acupuncture conducts its own impulse to the sensory center and prohibits conduction of pain impulse from viscera through the small A delta and C fibers which are located in a substantia gelatinosa of the spinal cord with the alpha and beta fibers.[4,47]

Acupuncture provides a certain degree of stimulation on the meridian points and reportedly uses the reactions of the autonomic nervous system to increase the healing power of the diseased body. Reflex therapy such as acupuncture, however, has not been well received in modern medicine. Acupuncture may be primarily effective for signs and symptoms which are not amenable to modern medical techniques by correcting a dysfunction of the autonomic nerve system.

TABLE III

1. *Diseases Hard to Cure*	2. *Discomfort of Diseases*	3. *Pain Clinic*
Asthma	Backache	Pain which is
Peptic Ulcer	Headache	not located on the
Spastic Colitis	Nasal Obstruction	direct nerve path
Nocturia	Constipation	Pain due to
Neurosis	Cough	metabolic
Migraine	Heartburn	disturbances
Hemiplegia	Singultus	Not severe
Meneire's Disease	Nausea, Vomiting	does not need
Essential Hypertension	Menstral Pain	nerve block
Diabetes Mellitus		(Post-op)
Dysmenorrhea		Patients do not
Allergy		want to have
Neurosis		block or allergic
Hysteria		
Sleeplessness		
Impotence		
Menopausal Disorders		
Myopia		
Deaf		
Epilepsy		
Cataract		

Possible Indications for Acupuncture

POSSIBLE INDICATIONS OF ACUPUNCTURE

Modern medicine as developed in the western hemisphere and now practiced throughout the world appears to be most effective in the cure of the diseased people. Modern medicine has accumulated an extensive amount of experimental and objective studies. However, there are certain conditions, diseases and symptom complexes in which modern medicine is neither indicated nor effective. These symptom complexes are the conditions which may be affected by acupuncture (Fig. 16 and Table III). These are:

1. Diseases which are presently incurable or difficult to treat.
2. Discomfort accompanying various diseases.
3. Pain (patients with chronic pain are becoming more of a problem for themselves, families and even the nation).

CHAPTER 2

CLINICAL PRACTICE OF ACUPUNCTURE

BASIC CLINICAL KNOWLEDGE OF PROCEDURES

Needle

There are many kinds of needles available. The size of the needles commonly used ranges from the diameter of a hair to that of a sewing needle. In China, round and cutting needles are commonly used and the sizes commonly employed vary from No. 26 to No. 32 (the smaller the number, the larger the diameter). Lengths of the needles ranges from 1.5 cm to 2.5 cm. In Japan, the size ranges from No. 0 to No. 10 (diameter of No. 0 is approximately 0.14 mm, No. 10, 0.34 mm and length ranges from 3 cm to 10 cm). In Europe, the needles are relatively shorter and slightly wider in diameter.

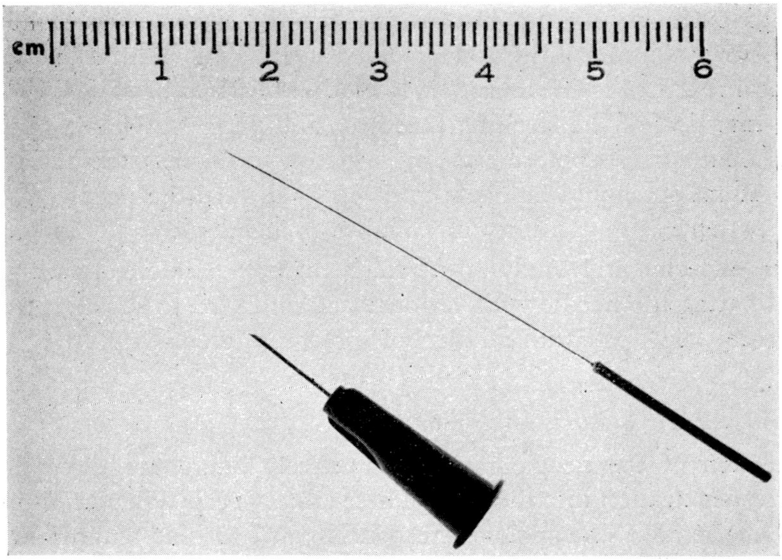

Figure 17: Size comparison of 25 gauge hypodermic needle at left and an acupuncture needle at right.

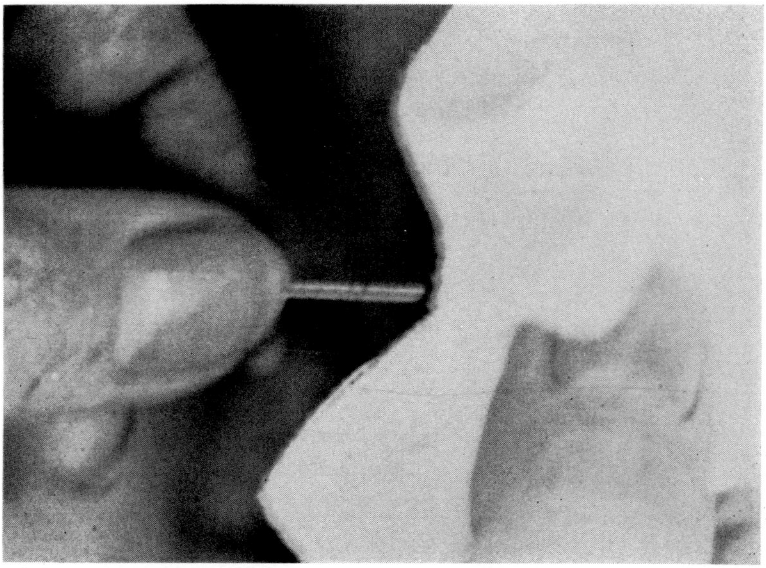

Figure 18: An acupuncture needle was contaminated with various bacteria (pseudomonas, kleubsiella, and E. coli) and wiped once with an alcohol sponge.

Needles are made of gold, silver, iron, platinum or stainless steel. The stainless steel needles are most commonly used at present. We use a stainless steel needle of 0.2 mm in diameter and 6 cm in length (Fig. 17). If the diameter is larger, then the patient may well feel some pain on application of the needle to a sensitive area of the body.

Infection due to needle puncture is said to be extremely rare. This may be due to the minor injury created by the needle being controlled by biological reaction at this area.[12] It is routine to wipe the skin with alcohol before insertion of the sterilized needle. The needle itself may be wiped with alcohol sponges before each insertion on the same patient. However, special attention should be made to carefully discard the needles following use in patients with a history of jaundice or hepatitis.

Our experimental study to attempt to isolate micro-organisms after contaminating the needle with various bacteria failed to show growth after the needle was wiped with an alcohol sponge (Figs. 18, 19).

Techniques of Needle Insertion

Insertion of the needle requires practice! There are three different angles of penetration into the skin. These are: 1—perpendicular, 2—oblique, and 3—horizontal. The angles correspond to 90°, 45° and a minimum angle respectively. These may be chosen on the basis of thickness of skin and proximity to muscle or bone at the desired puncture point. Depth of pene-

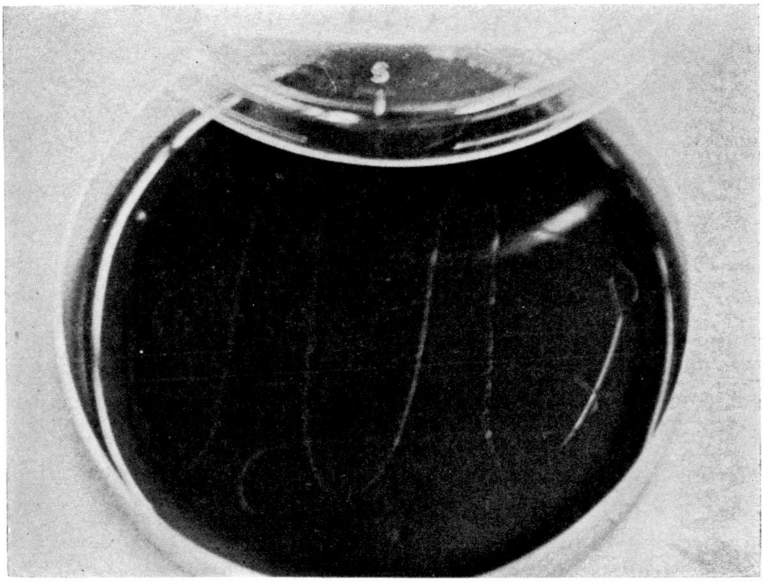

Figure 19: No organism was isolated from this needle by culture.

tration will vary with an average of 10, 30, and 40 mm at head, shoulder and back regions respectively.

Methods of Insertion

TAPPING METHOD (TUBE METHOD): This is the simplest method for beginners (Fig. 20). When the diameter of the needle is small, this method

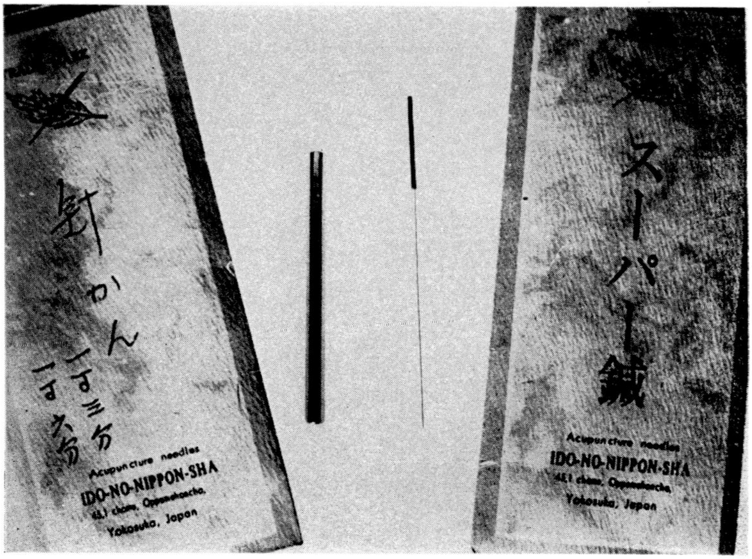

Figure 20: Acupuncture needle and tube.

is extremely effective. Place the needle into the tube from either direction. The tube is shorter than the needle by 5 mm or more. The above step can be done with practice by one hand and this, then, is called the one-hand method. Briefly massage the area where the needle is to be placed with left thumb or index finger (Fig. 21). Next place the tube perpendicularly on the acupuncture point by holding it between left thumb and index finger (Fig. 22). Be certain the needle tip is not outside the tube since this is more painful. Compress the tube gently against the skin with the left fingers fixing the tube against it. Finally, gentle tapping of the needle handle with the right index finger introdues the needle quite easily. The tapping finger must be removed from the needle head immediately after tapping; otherwise, it creates pain (Fig. 23). Remove the tube gently with the left fingers (Fig. 24). The needle may be pushed into the muscle with the right index finger and thumb. If the muscle contracts while holding the needle in position, wait a short period or massage the area around the needle. If not successful in moving the needle, then apply a second needle with gentle force. If the needle bends, relax and wait to advance it.

TWIRLING METHOD (FREE-HAND METHOD): Contact the left thumb and

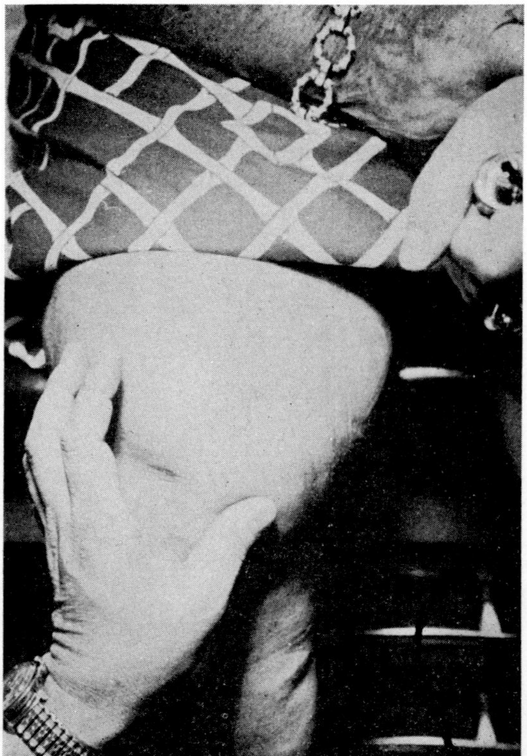

Figure 21: Massage the area where the needle is to be placed.

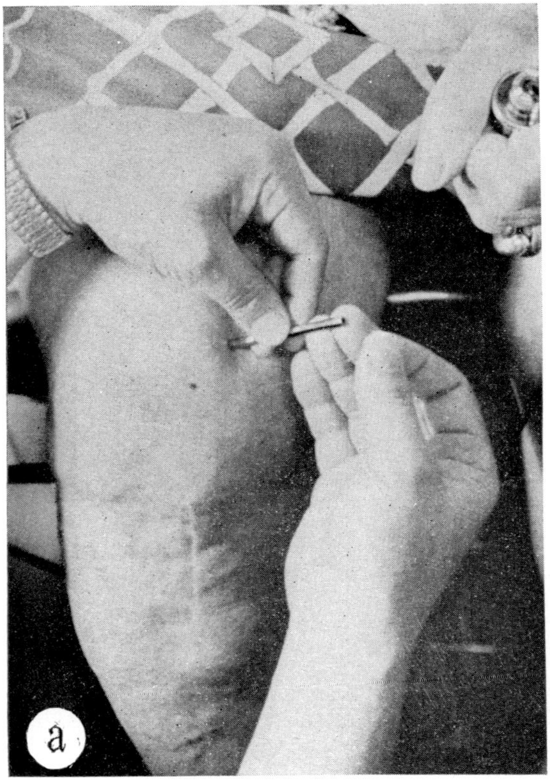

Figure 22: Place the tube perpendicularly on the acupuncture point by holding it between the left thumb and index finger. (a) knee area, (b) gluteal area.

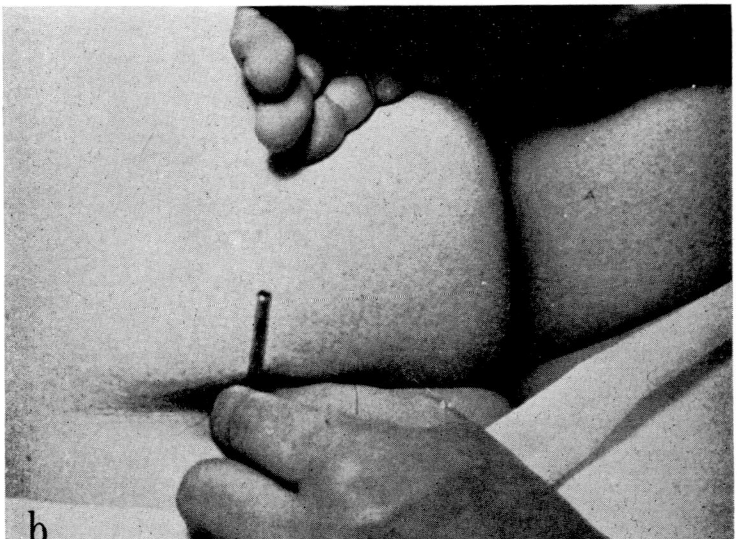

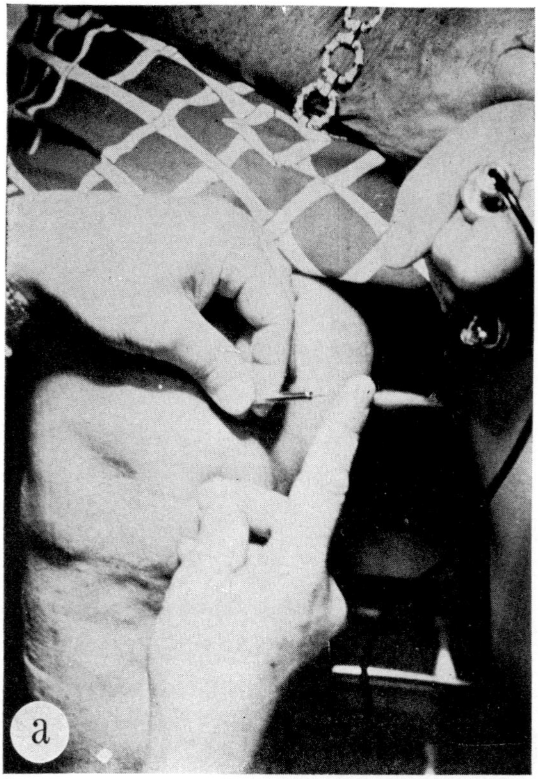

Figure 23: Place the needle inside the tube. Then, tap the needle head with the right index finger: (a) knee area; (b) arm area.

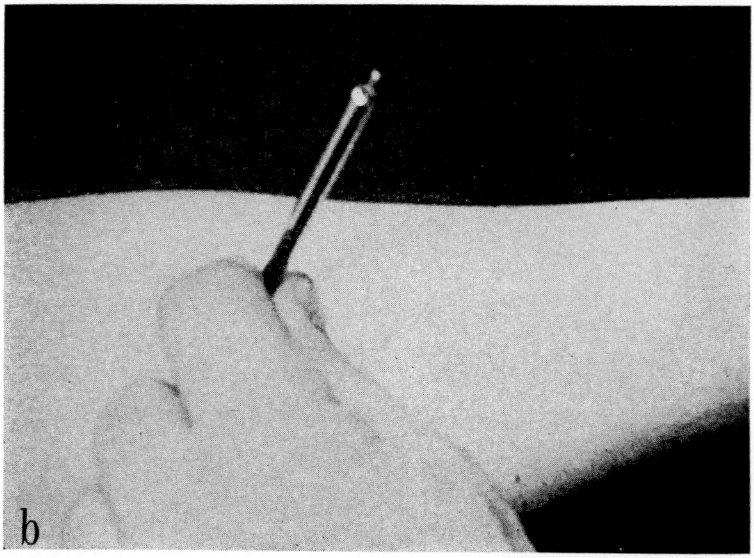

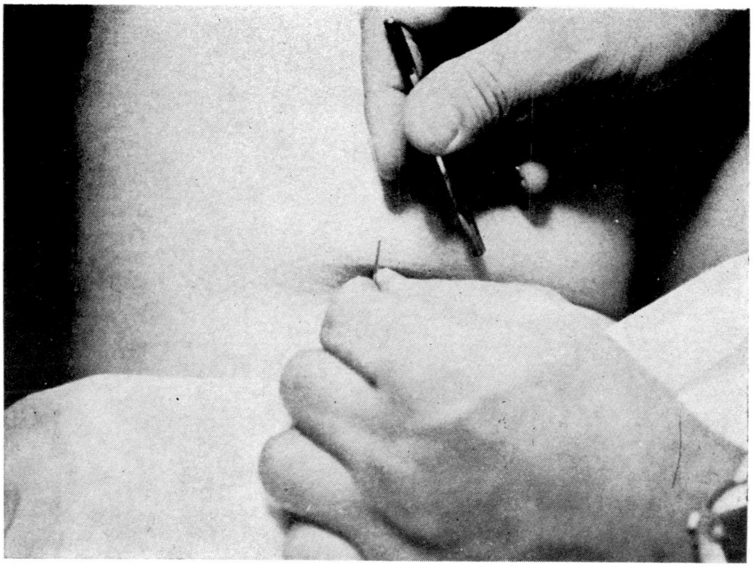

Figure 24: Remove the tube; the needle is now inserted.

index finger at the acupuncture point. This hand is called the *pushing hand* (Fig. 25). Next, the motion is skin cutting with the needle tip which is followed by insertion of the needle by pushing and twirling the needle by the right hand (Figs. 26, 27). It is essential not to push too hard with the *pushing hand*. Very light contact of the pushing hand to the skin is the key.

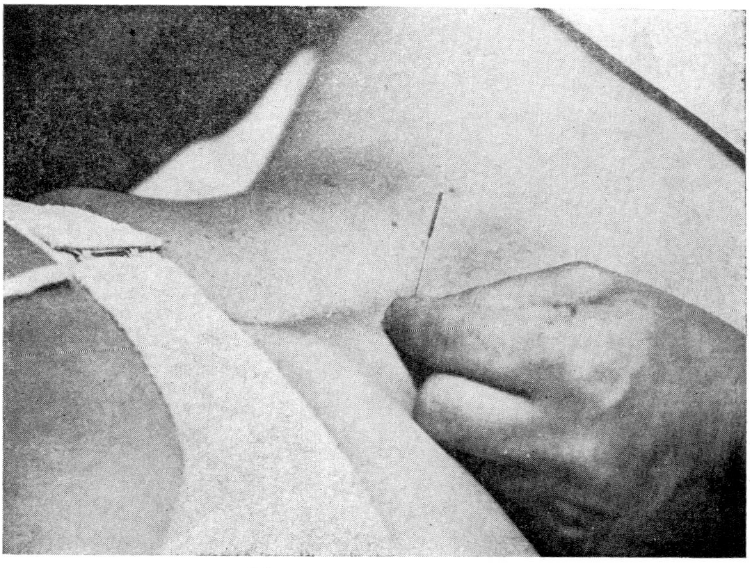

Figure 25: *Pushing Hand* at the acupuncture point.

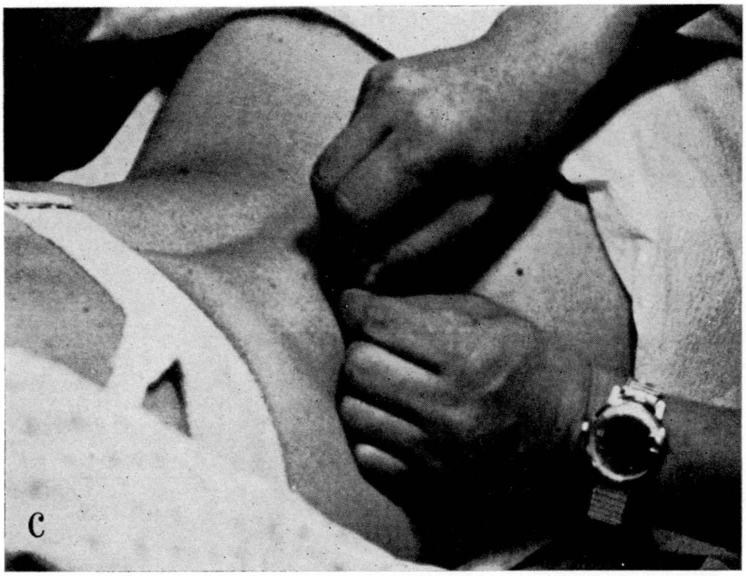

Figure 26: Pushing and twirling of the needle by the right hand penetrates the needle into the skin.

If the skin is pushed harder with the pushing hand, the skin tone is increased and thus resists the needle's insertion.

USE OF ACUPUNCTURE NEEDLE HOLDER: The needle is placed into the needle holder which allows the plunger to move the needle up and down

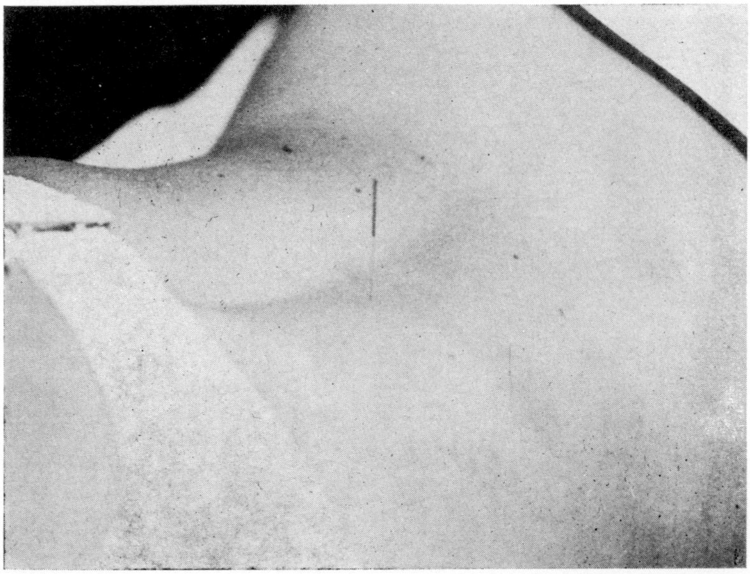

Figure 27: Needle is now inserted at the acupuncture point.

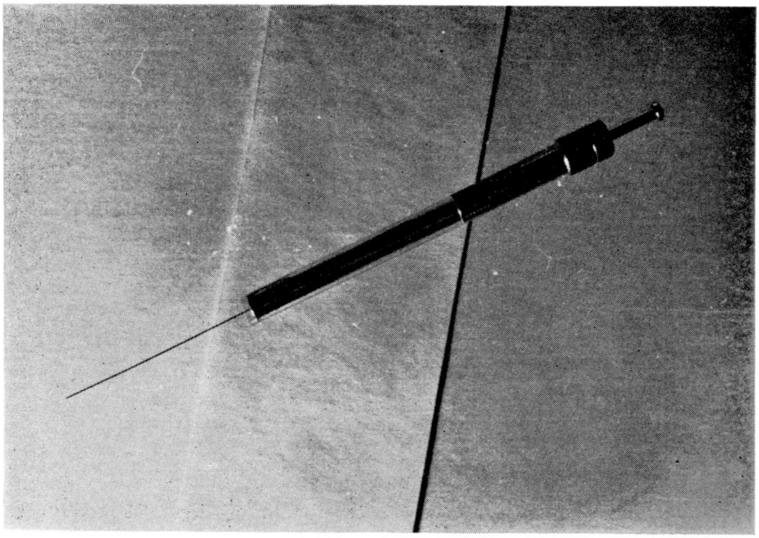

Figure 28: Acupuncture needle holder.

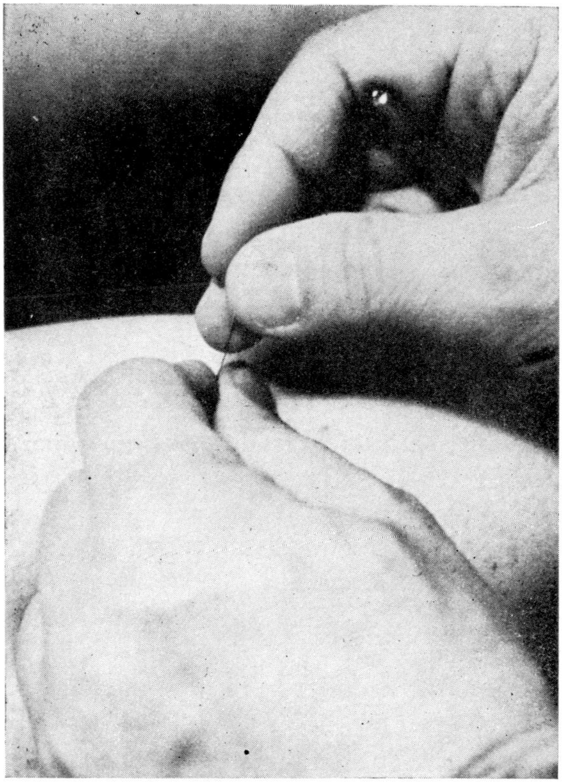

Figure 29: Twirling

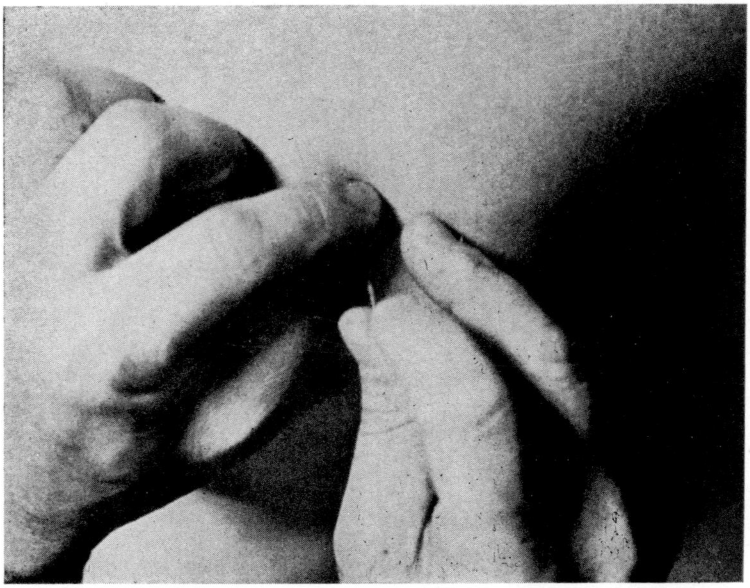

Figure 30: Sparrow pecking motion.

to an exact preset distance (Fig. 28). This apparatus is ideal for placebo effect of acupuncture in experimental study.

Advancement of Needle and Needle Motion

The objective of this is to create *needle feeling* in the patient. This is a dull, aching, paralyzing or compressing feeling or combination of these sensations that radiates to a distal or proximal portion of the body. When the patient notices the *needle feeling* then the operator should increase the feeling by various needle motions. Numerous motions are available. The major motions are as follows:

1. *Single Stick:* Insert the needle to a certain depth and remove.
2. *Twirling:* Twirl the needle during an in and out motion. This is a relatively strong stimulation (Fig. 29).
3. *Sparrow-pecking:* Insert the needle in to a certain depth then move up and down rapidly. The faster motion causes strong stimulation (Fig. 30).
4. *Vibration:* Insert a needle into a certain depth and vibrate the needle head by hitting gently with the finger.
5. *Intermittent:* Insert a needle, then wait before further advancement. This stimulation is considered mild.
6. *Retention Method:* Leave a needle in the cutis for 5 to 20 minutes. The skin around the needle becomes hyperemic (Fig. 31).
7. *Contact Method:* Instead of inserting needle, contact the needle

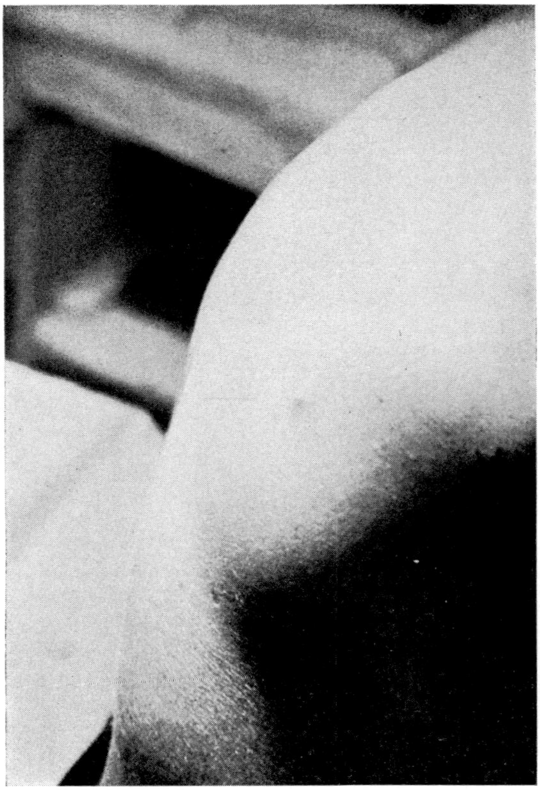

Figure 31: Retention method.

handle to the acupuncture point. This provides light stimulation and is often used in pediatric practice.

Pre and Post Acupuncture Massage

In order to prepare the body for acceptance of needle stimulation, light massage over skin and muscle are recommended. Pre-puncture massage makes skin cutting easier and makes the patient relax. In addition to these advantages, it may detect pathology such as nodules, spasm, pain, and depression. Post-puncture massage may help to confirm hypersenitivity of muscle and confirm disappearance of pain or hard nodules which existed before the acupuncture.

Electric Acupuncture

Instead of hand manipulation of the needle, electric current may be used as a method of stimulation.

After placing the needle at the point, 200 microamperes, 6 to 12 volts of electric current is given for 10 seconds. Sparrow pecking may be added at one per second while applying electricity (Fig. 32). Prior to the removal of the needle, the electric current should be disconnected in order to prevent pain.

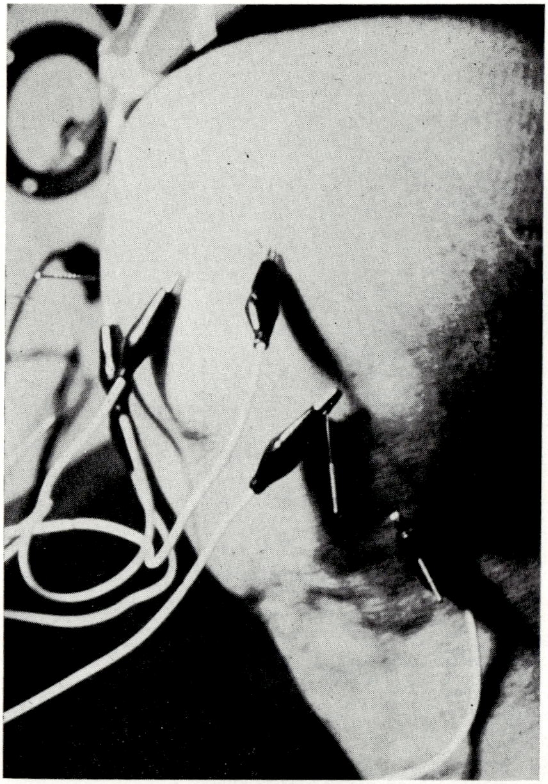

Figure 32: Neurometer in use. We do not know the exact resistance of the body; therefore, the current introduced into the point is not exactly 200 microamperes. However, it is possible to measure the body resistance using a known resistor.

Duration of Acupuncture and Interval

The amount of stimulation = (strength of stimulation) × (number of treatments); this is dependent on the sensitivity of the patient. The same person may change sensitivity on a different day. Gradual increases of stimulation is essential. In general, for acute disease, treatment should be given once a day for ten days and then held for three to seven days. For chronic ailments treatment is given once every two to three days for ten treatments and then held for seven days.

Position of Patients

Lying, sitting, supine, prone or side position may be used. Whichever is easier for the patient and physician is appropriate. A special position, however, may be needed in order to relax the painful area (Fig. 33 a to j).

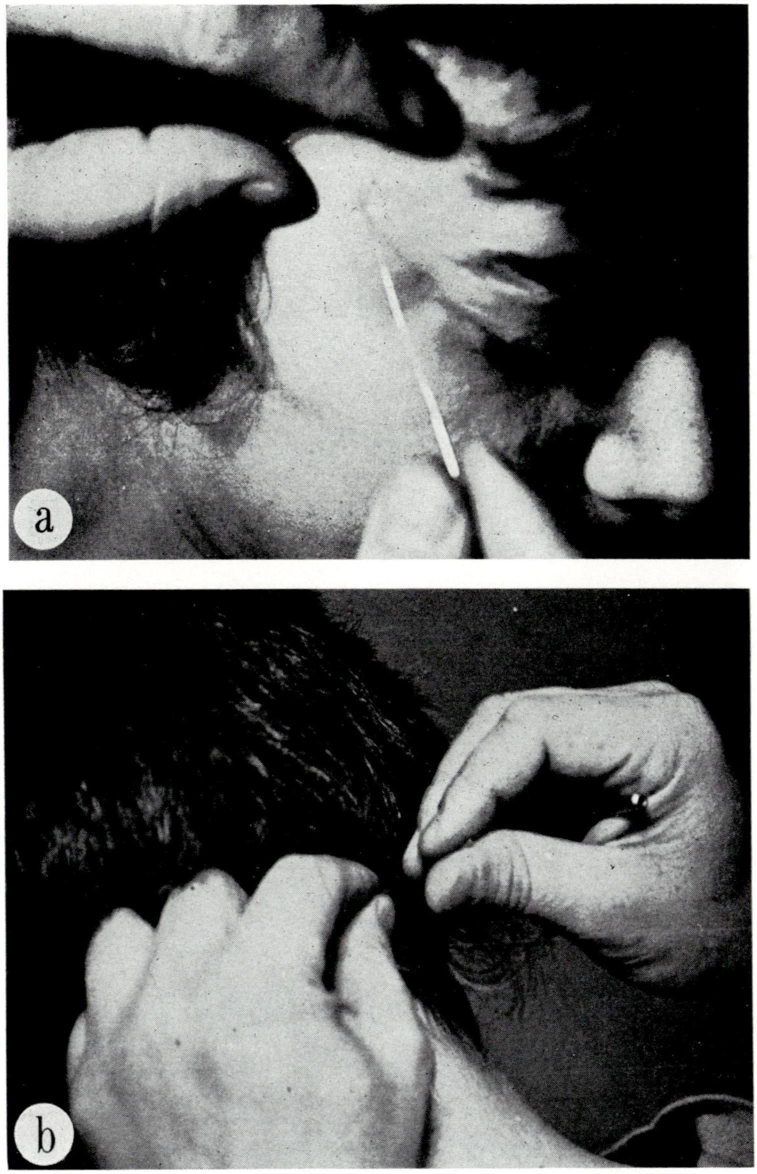

Figure 33: POSITIONS OF PATIENT. (a and b) Sitting position.

Complications

DIZZINESS: Stop acupuncture and use conservative treatment. If it is not improved and unconsciousness develops, compress the point at *Jinchiyu* or *Sanri*. To prevent this complication do not use acupuncture when the patient is hungry or exhausted. For the initial acupuncture, use light stimulation.

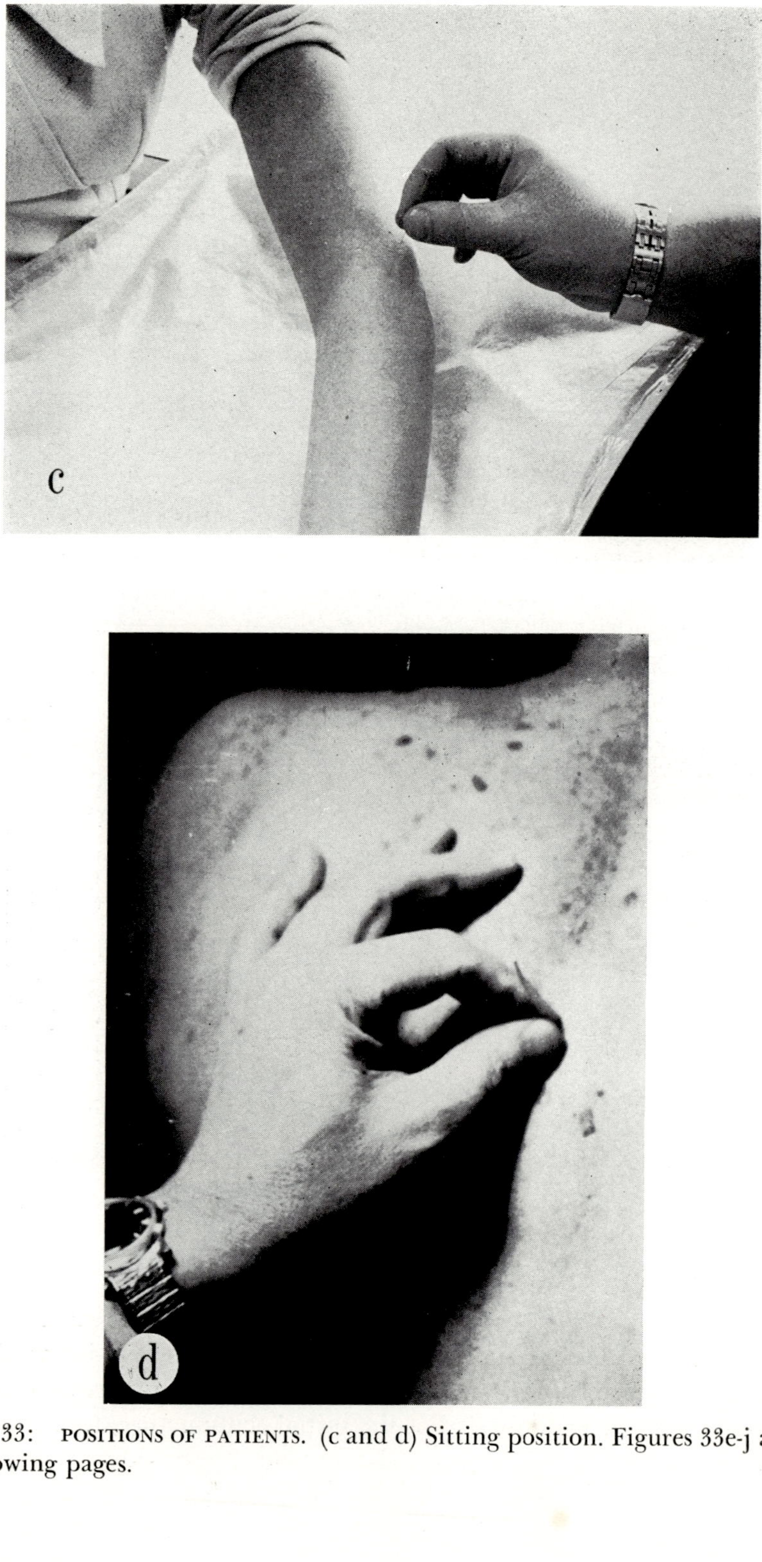

Figure 33: POSITIONS OF PATIENTS. (c and d) Sitting position. Figures 33e-j appear on following pages.

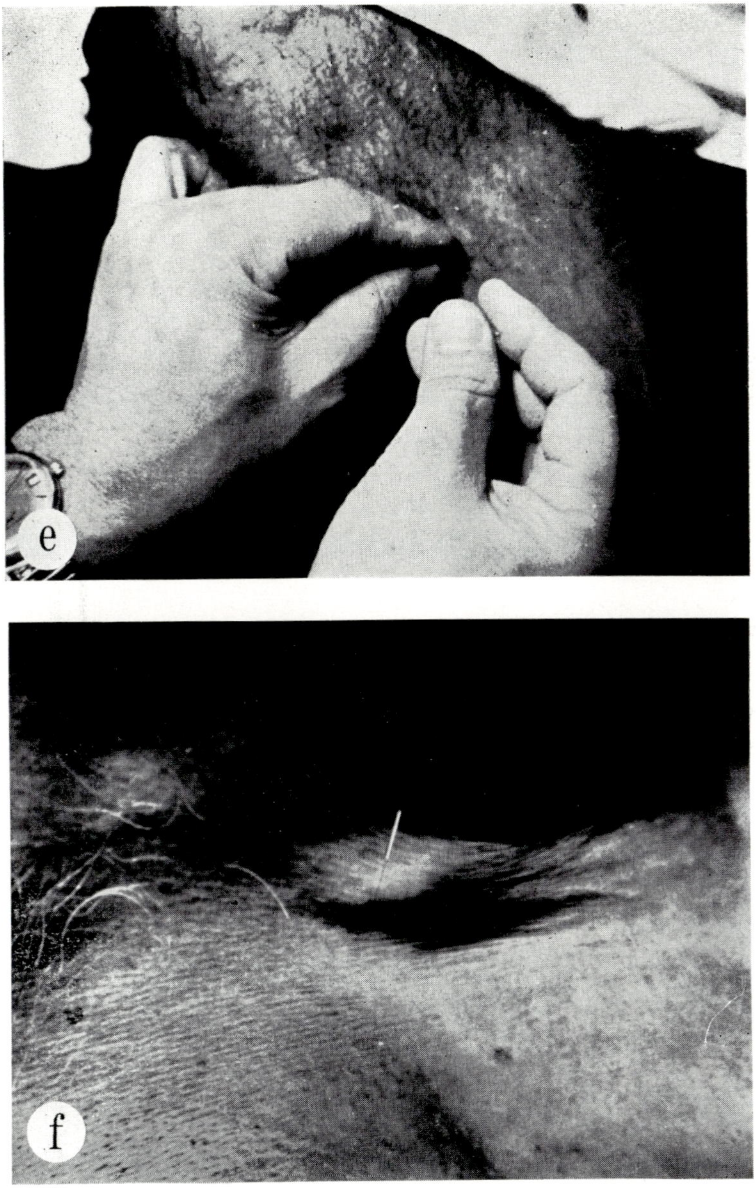

Figure 33: POSITIONS OF PATIENT. (e) Sitting position. (f) Supine position.

Preparation of Needle

The needles are very small and easily damaged. A damaged needle causes unnecessary pain at the time of the acupuncture. Therefore, they should be kept in a supportive holder until used in treatment. Careful observation of the needle is essential. If the needle tip becomes dull, use fine grain sandpaper and wipe the needle with the sandpaper. Microscopic

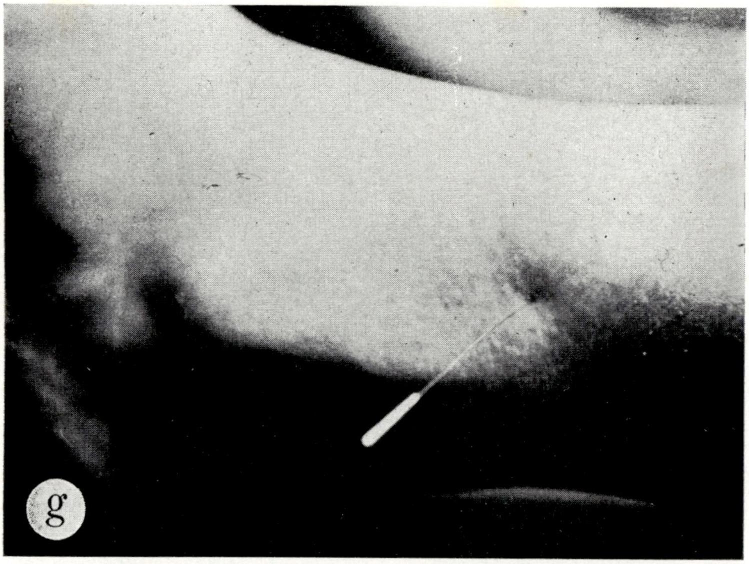

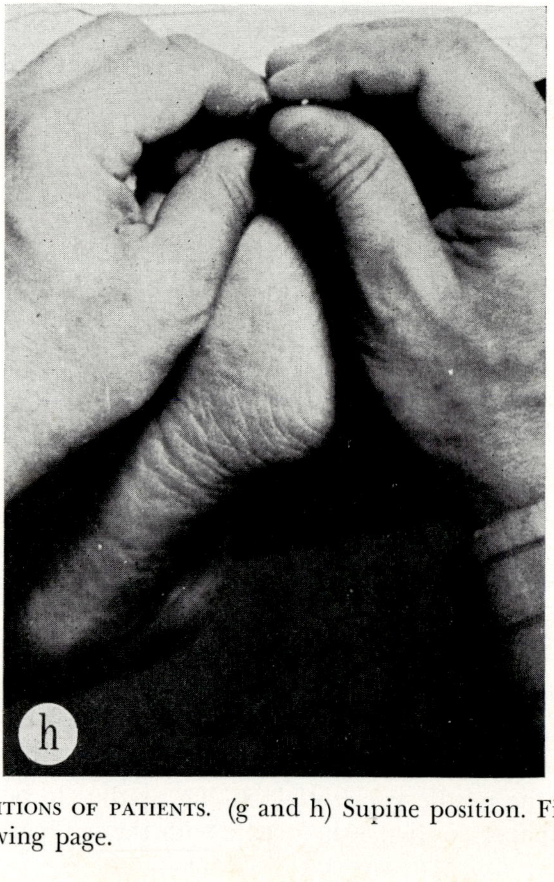

Figure 33: POSITIONS OF PATIENTS. (g and h) Supine position. Figure 33 i and j appear on following page.

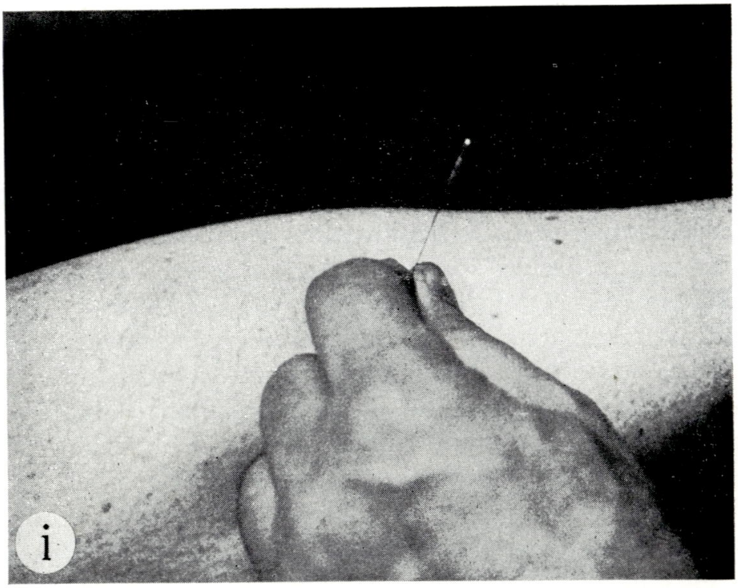

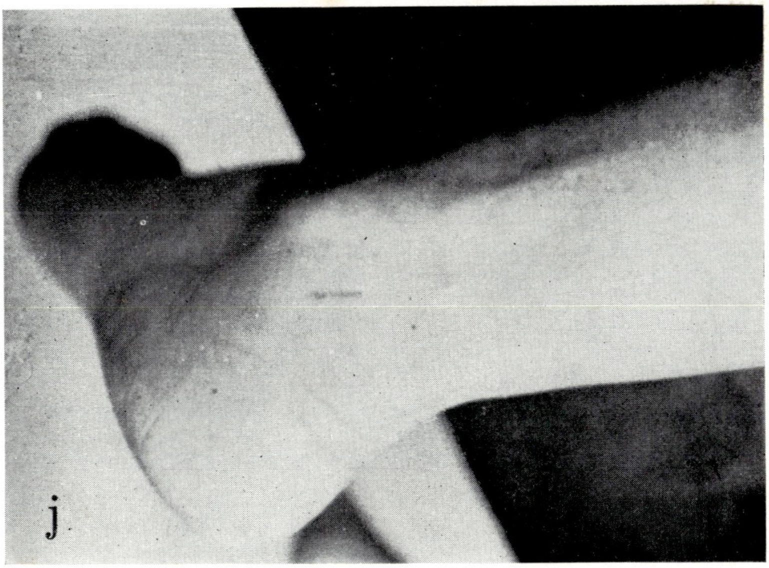

Figure 33: POSITIONS OF PATIENTS. (i and j) Prone position.

observation with a 50 x eyepiece is helpful in identifying characteristics of the used needle. When the needle is bent, place the needle between two cardboard pieces and manipulate until straight.

ACUPUNCTURE POINTS

How to Locate and Insert Needles

General

One of the most important factors to be considered in effective acupuncture is accurate selection of acupuncture points. These points must be selected according to the specific points for the specific ailment.

In order to describe the acupuncture points, certain factors should be observed.

Mark skin grossly according to the text (Figs. 34, and Plate I). The names of these acupuncture points are originally written in Chinese and they represent efficacy, anatomical distribution, shape of the region, or meridian function. This makes it difficult for English speaking physicians to memorize such names. Accordingly, special effort has been made to standardize these points by utilizing alphabetic and numeric coordinates. This has been without uniform success.

Place your finger on the area and compress. Usually you will find elastic muscle fiber and a small indented area. This area is usually tender and thought to be a meridian point (acupuncture point) (Fig. 21).

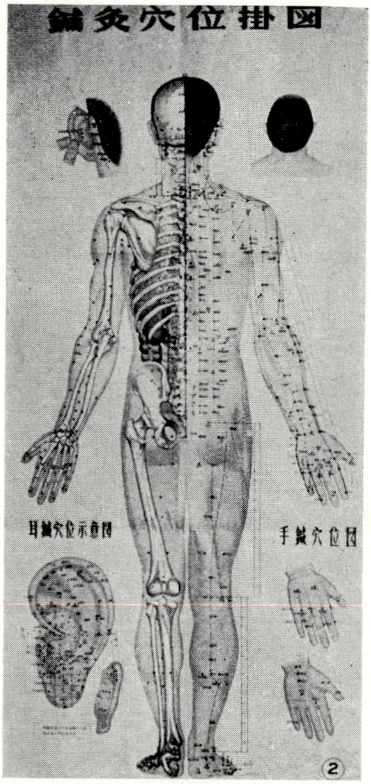

Figure 34: Acupuncture point (original).

PLATES 1a, 1b, 1c,

The selected acupuncture points

by this author

and their English names

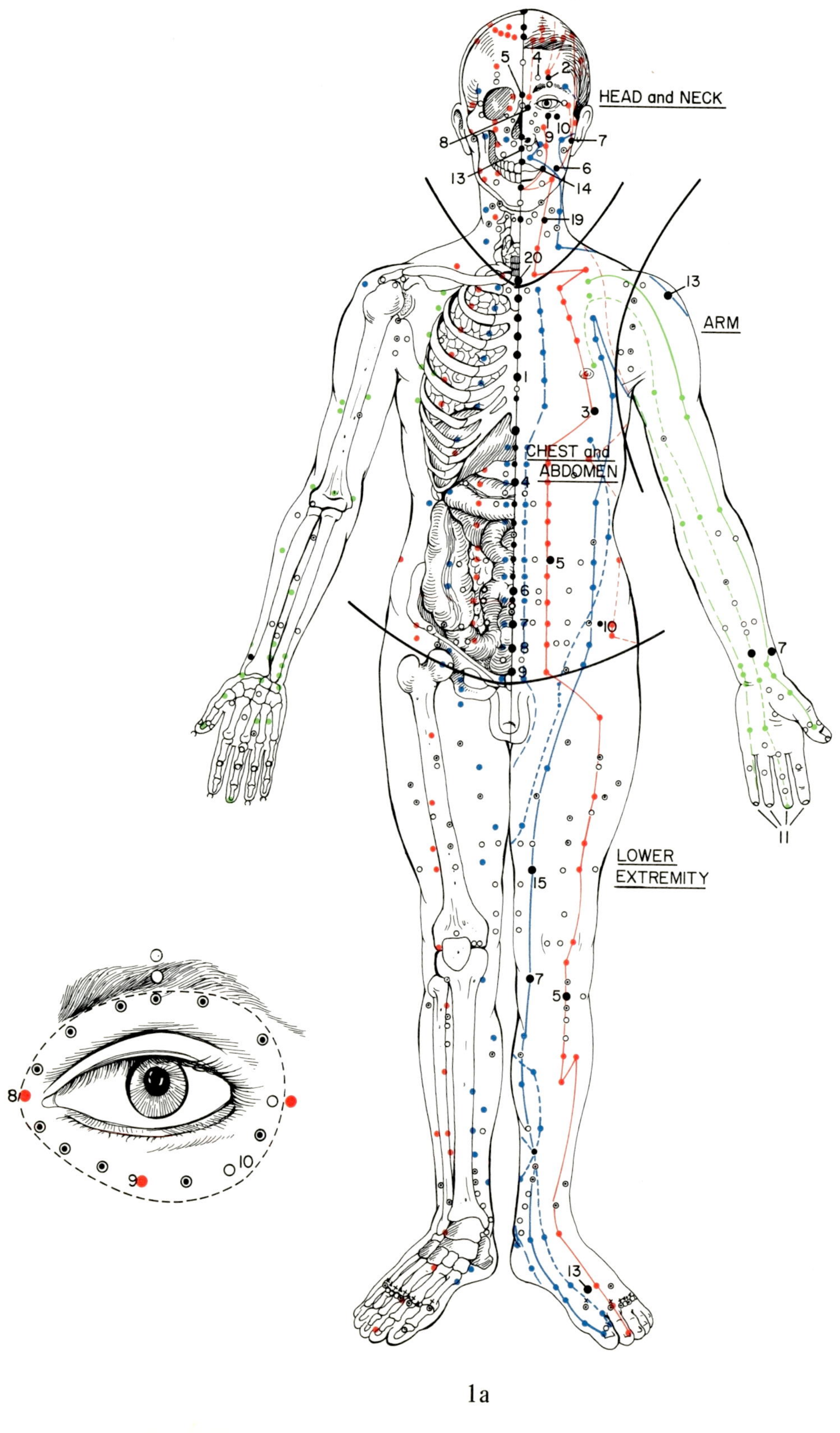
HEAD and NECK
ARM
CHEST and
ABDOMEN
LOWER
EXTREMITY
5
4
2
9
10
8
7
13
6
14
19
20
13
1
3
4
5
6
7
8
9
10
7
11
15
7
5
13
8
9
10

1a

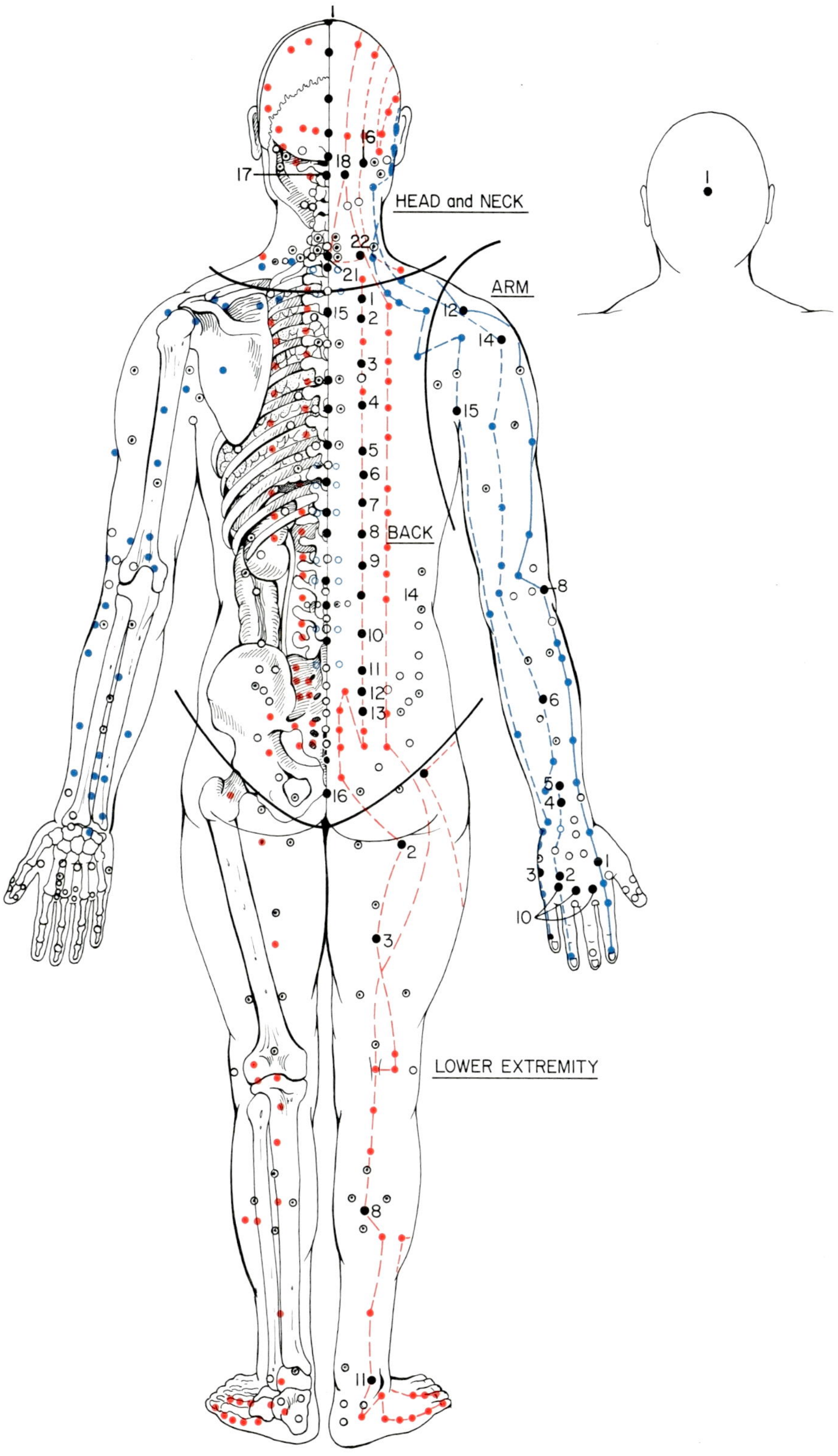
HEAD and NECK
ARM
BACK
LOWER EXTREMITY

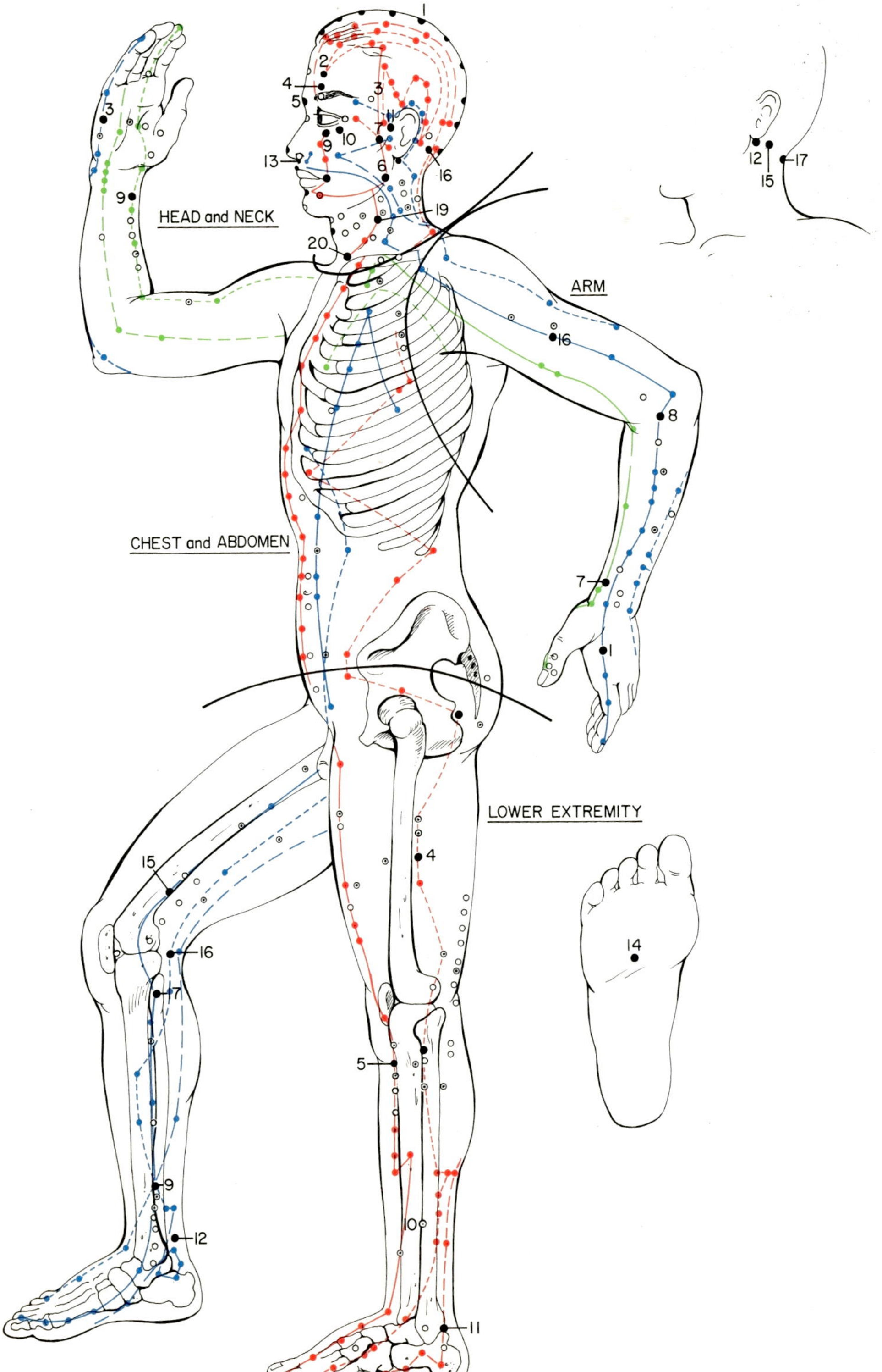
HEAD and NECK
ARM
CHEST and ABDOMEN
LOWER EXTREMITY
1
2
3
4
5
7
9
10
11
13
6
16
19
20
3
9
12
15
17
16
8
7
1
4
15
16
17
9
12
5
10
11
14

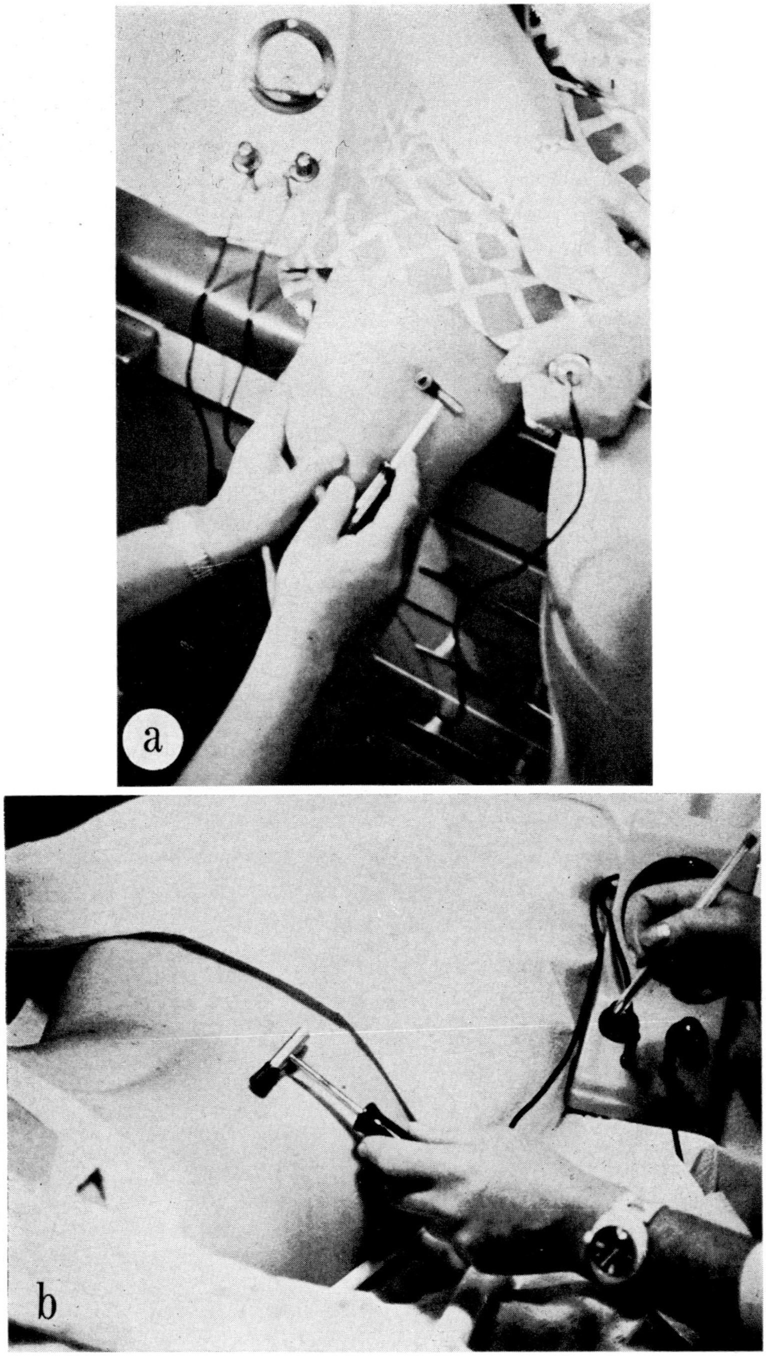

Figure 35: Measurement of electrosensitive points (a and b). It is essential that the detecting electrode should be placed on the skin with a constant pressure and constant period. A device has been made to read the pressure applied on the skin.

Recent advancement in acupuncture necessitates measurement of the electric activity of the skin. Electro-permeability or sensitivity of the skin is measured using a neurometer set at 12 volts. (Electropermeable or sensitive points may be considered as the points where skin resistance is low). Many meridian points are electropermeable or sensitive points (Fig. 35).

I have selected seventy of the most common and effective points based upon various acupuncture textbooks including the most recent, popular, Chinese textbook and provided new English names for every point (Plate I).

These points are not only useful for acupuncture but could be used for any stimulation methods. These include electric acupuncture application, metallic ball, finger pressure and application of other special stimulation therapy. But this paper provides only the most commonly used indications. Intelligent utilization of these points for stimulation therapy may not only be effective for control of pain, but also useful for preventive medicine.

INDEX OF SELECTED POINTS

Head and Neck

1. Vertex	hyakue, pai hui (GV20)
2. Supraorbital	yohaku, yang-pei (GB14)
3. Temporal	taiyo, tai-yang
4. Mid-eyebrow	bichiyu, chien
5. Glabella	Indo, yin-tang
6. Inferior Masseter	kyoshiya, chia-che (S3)
7. Infratemporal	Gekan, hsia-kuan (S2)
8. Median canthus	seimei, chang-ming (B1)
9. Midinfraorbital	shiyokyu, cheng-chi (S4)
10. Lateral infraorbital	kyugo, chiu-hon
11. Superior tragus	jimon, erh-men (T21)
12. Posterior earlobe	eifu, I-feng (T17)
13. Infranasal	jinchiyu, jen-chung (L1)
14. Lateral oral angle	chiso, ti-ts'ang (S7)
15. Inframastoid	Imei I-mong
16. High lateral trapezius	Fuchi, fengs-chi (GB31)
17. C1-C2	Amon, ya-men (GV15)
18. Para C1-C2	Tenchyu, tien-chu (B10)
19. Lateral thyroid	jingei jen-ying (S9)
20. Supra Sternal	tentotsu, t'ien-t'u (CV22)
21. C7-T1	Daizui, ta-ch'ui (GV14)
22. Para C7-T1	Chizen

Chest and Abdomen

1. Midsternum	danchyu, shan-chung (CV17)
2. Subxyphoid	kyubi (chiu-wei (CV15)
3. Sub Breast	nyukon, Ju-keng (S18)
4. Midepigastrium	chyukan, chung-wuan (CV12)
5. Lateral umbilicus	tensu, t'ien-shu (S25)
6. Upper hypogastrium	kikai, chi-hai (CV)
7. Low hypogastrium	kangen, kuan-yuan (CV4)
8. Lower hypogastrium	chyu kyoku, chung-chi (CV3)
9. Suprapubic	kyoku kotsu chu-ku (CV2)
10. Lateral inguinal	Iho

Back

1. para T2-T3	fumon, feng-men (B12)
2. para T3-T4 (lung)	haiyu, fei-yu (B13)
3. para T5-T6 (heart)	shinyu, hsin-yu (B16)
4. para T7-T8 (diaphragm)	kakuyu, ke-yu (B17)
5. para T9-T10 (liver)	kanyu, kenye (B18)
6. para T10-T11 (gallbladder)	tanyu, tanyu (B19)
7. para T11-T12 (spleen)	hiyu, p'i-yu (B20)
8. para T12-L1 (stomach)	Iyu, wei-yu (B21)
9. para L2-L3 (kidney)	jinyu, shen-yu (B23)
10. para L4-L5 (colon)	daichyoyu, ta-chang-yu (B25)
11. para L5-S1	Kangenyu kuan-yuan-yu (B26)
12. para S1-S2 (small bowel)	shyochyoyu, hsiao-ch'ang-yu (B27)
13. para S2-S3 (bladder)	bokoyu, p'ang-k'uang-yu (B28)
14. Lateral L2-L3	shishitsu chih-shih (B47)
15. T3-T4	mumei
16. Posterior anal	chyokyo, ch'ang-ch'iang (GV 1)

Upper Extremities

1. First dorsal web	gokoku, ho-ku (L14)
2. Fourth dorsal web	chyushyo, chung-chu (T3)
3. Fifth lateral metacarpal	kokei, hou-chi (SI3)
4. Dorsal distal forearm	gaikan, waikuan (T5)
5. Dorsal low forearm	shiko, chih-kou (T6)
6. Dorsal upper forearm	shitoku szu-tu (T9)
7. Radial styloid process	letsuketsu, lieh-ch'uen (L7)
8. Lateral cubital crease	kyokuchi, chu-ch'ih (LI11)
9. Volar distal forearm	naikan, neikuan (P6)
10. Inter M.P. joint	hachija, pa-hsieh
11. Finger tip	jissen, shih-hsuan

12. Claviculo scapular junction	kyokotsu, chu-ku (LI16)
13. Anterior acromion	kengu, chien-yu (LI15)
14. Posterior acromion	kenko, chien-liao (T14)
15. Posterior axillary crease	kentei, chien-chen (SI9)
16. Midlateral humerus	pi-nao (LI14)

Lower Extremities

1. Posterior trochanter	kanchyo, huan-tiao (GB30)
2. Midgluteal crease	shiyofu, ch'eng-fu (B50)
3. Posterior midthigh	yinmon, yin-men (B51)
4. Lateral midthigh	fui chi, fongchih (GB20)
5. Lateral upper tibia	ashi-sanri, tsu-san-li (S36)
6. Anterior upper fibula	yoryosen, yang-lin-chuan (GB34)
7. Upper posterior tibia	inryosen, yin-lin-ch'uan (SP9)
8. Mid-Gastrocnemius	shyozan, ch'eng-san (B57)
9. Posterior low tibia	saninko, san-yin-chiao (SP6)
10. Anterior lower fibula	zetsukotsu, chueh-ku
11. Posterior lateral malleolus	konron, kun-chun (B60)
12. Posterior medial malleolus	taikei, tai-chi (K3)
13. First metatarsal	taishiyo, t'ai-ch'ung (LV3)
14. Sole of foot	yosen, yung-ch'uan (K1)
15. Median supra patella	ketsukai, hsueh-hai (SP10)
16. Median popliteal crease	kyokusen, chu-chuan (LV8)

SPECIFIC POINTS (HOW TO SELECT)

Head and Neck

1. Vertex (Hyakue, pai-hui) Figure 36.
   a. Intersection of imaginary interaural line between upper portion of two ears and middle sagittal line.

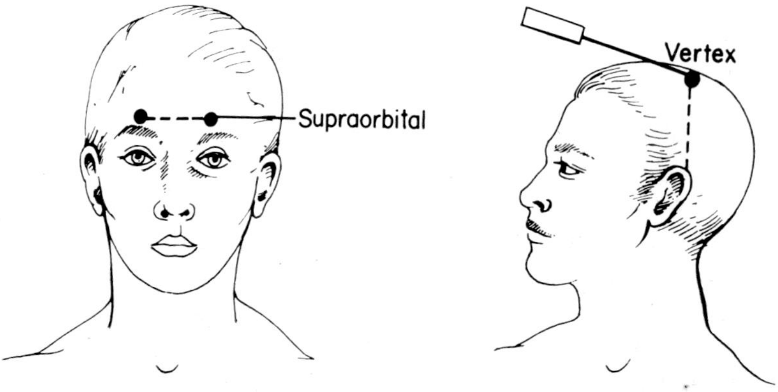

Figure 36: Supraorbital and Vertex.

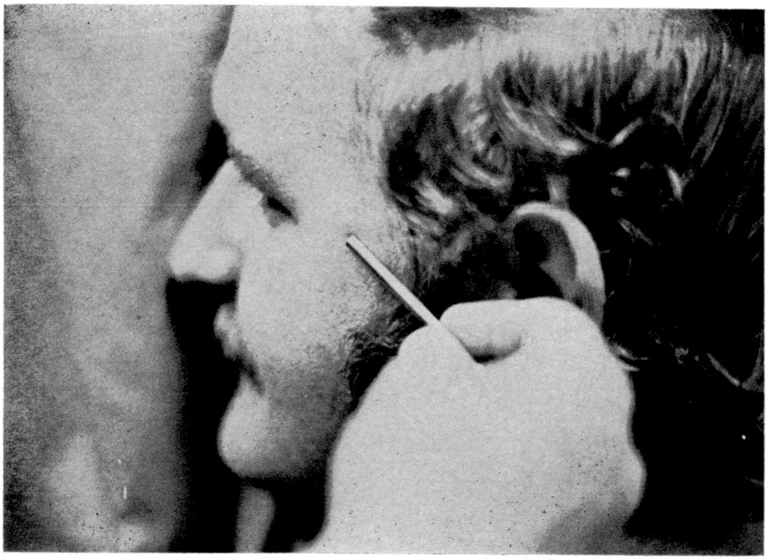

Figure 37: Temporal.

b. Horizontal stick to a depth of one inch.
c. Radiate to entire head.
d. Headache, hypertension, insomnia.
e. Caution: In infants, fontanelle is open and therefore dangerous.

2. Supraorbital (Yohaku, Yang-pe) Figure 36.
    a. One fingerbreadth upward from the mid-portion of eyebrow.
    b. Horizontal stick down to mid-eyebrow.
    c. Pressure pain locally.
    d. Facial paralysis, nystagmus, frontal headache.
3. Temporal (Taiyo, Tai-yang) Figure 37.

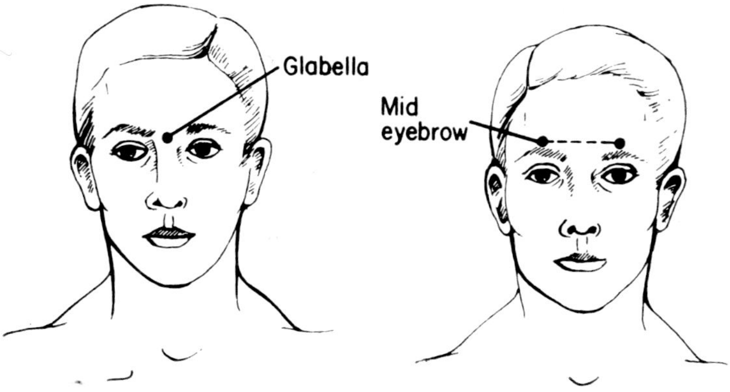

Figure 38: Glabella, mid-eyebrow.

a. One fingerbreadth lateral from between corner of eyebrow and eye.
b. Direct stick 0.5 inch or oblique stick one inch aiming over the ear.
c. Pressure feeling radiated to the head.
d. Migraine, facial paralysis, eye diseases.
e. Caution: Potential damage to facial nerve.

4. Mid-Eyebrow (Bichiyu, chien) Figure 38
   a. Upper edge of eyebrow at middle portion.
   b. Pull skin between fingers and stick medially for one inch.
   c. Pressure feeling over eyebrow.
   d. Myopia, migraine, conjunctivitis.
5. Glabella (between eyebrows) (Indo, yin-tang) Figure 38.
   a. Between eyebrow just above nasion.
   b. Pull skin between fingers and insert needle inferiorly for one inch.
   c. Locally radiates dull pressure sensation.
   d. Frontal headache, rhinitis, eyepain, dizziness.
6. Inferior Masseter (Kyoshiya, Chia-che) Figure 39.
   a. One fingerbreadth anterior and superior of the mandibular angle over the massetor muscle.
   b. Oblique stick toward angle of mouth for one inch.
   c. Radiate to cheek.
   d. Dental pain, facial paralysis, mumps.
7. Infratemporal (Gekan, hsia-kuan) Figure 39.
   a. Infratemporal fossa, in front of earlobe.
   b. Direct stick for 0.5 inches or horizontal.
   c. Radiate the lateral half of the face.
   d. Dental pain, mandibular joint pain.
   e. Caution: potential damage to branches of facial nerve.
8. Median Canthus (Seimei, ching-ming) Figure 40.
   a. Internal edge of orbital bone at just above median canthus.

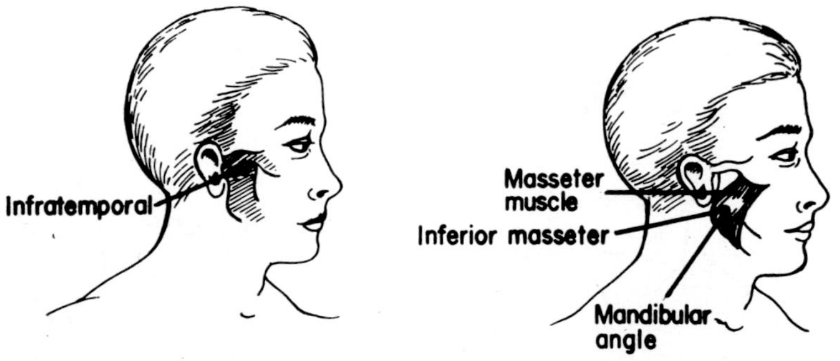

Figure 39: Infratemporal, inferior masseter.

b. Deep stick 0.5 inches deep.
c. Local pain with tears after removal of needle.
d. Eye disorders.
e. Caution: Avoid lacrimal duct.

9. Mid-infraorbital (Shiyo kyu, cheng chi) Figure 40.
   a. Between orbit and eyeball at midpoint of infraorbital ridge.
   b. Oblique stick just below the point toward median canthus.
   c. Pain and pressure to eyeball.
   d. Disease of eye including myopia.

10. Lateral infraorbital (Kyugo, Chiu-hon) Figure 41.
    a. Between eyeball and orbit one-third from the lateral border of the eyelid to medial border.
    b. Compress eyeball gently upward with left index finger and place needle one inch aiming posterior center of eyeball (optic nerve).
    c. Pain and pressure on eyeball.
    d. Hard to see (glaucoma, optic neuritis, optic nerve atrophy, retinal hemorrhage, conjuctivitis strabismus.

11. Superior tragus (Jimon, erh-men) Triple Figure 41.
    a. Superior anterior portion of the tragus.
    b. Open mouth. Perpendicular stick two inches deep.
    c. Radiate to ear and face.
    d. Tinnitis, deafness, ear disorders.

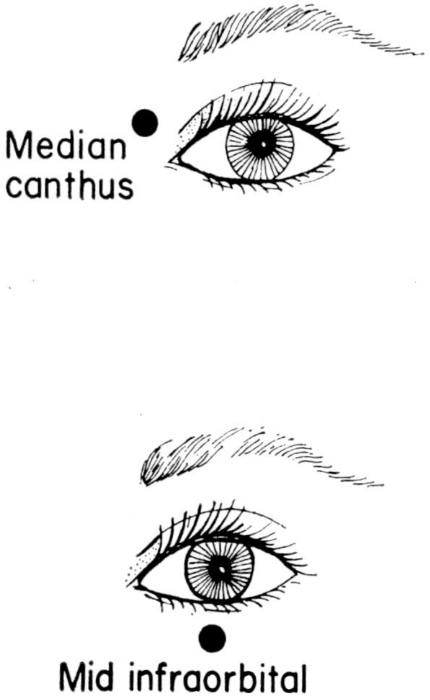

Figure 40: Median canthus, Mid-infraorbital.

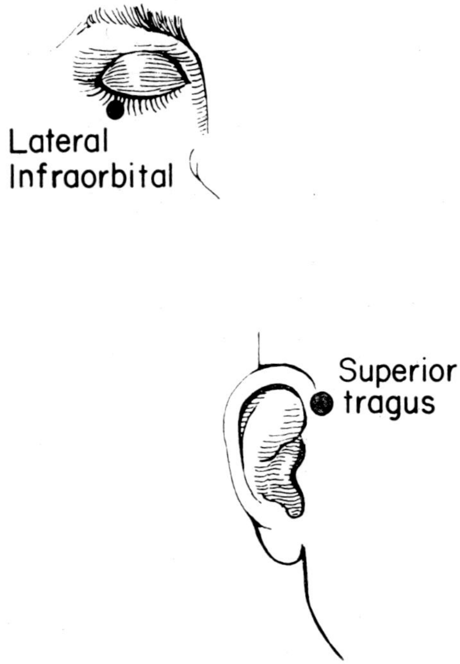

Figure 41: Lateral infraorbital, Superior tragus.

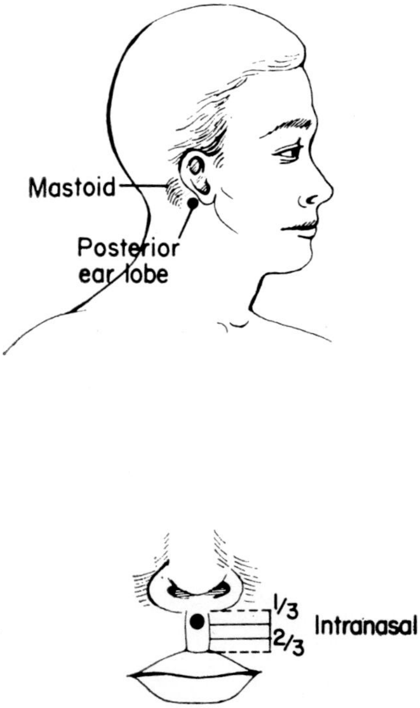

Figure 42: Posterior ear lobe, Infranasal.

12. Posterior Earlobe (Eifu, I-feng) Figure 42.
    a. Groove between earlobe and mastoid.
    b. Oblique stick at the surface of bone aiming at opposite ear.
    c. Radiate pressure pain to ear and temporal area.
    d. Deafness, dental pain, tinnitus, otorrhea.
13. Infranasal (jinchiyu, Jen-chung) Extra Meridian Figure 42.
    a. One third of distance from anterior nasal spine to midpoint of upper lip.
    b. Oblique stick one inch superiorly or one inch oblique stick transversely to left or right.
    c. Local pressure.
    d. Syncope, backache, severe heart and abdominal pain, diabetes, rhinitis, edema of face, tremor of lips.
14. Lateral Oral Angle (Chiso, ti-ts'ang) Gastric Meridian Figure 43.
    a. Half fingerbreadth lateral from the corner of the mouth.
    b. Horizontal stick needle one inch to *inferior masseter.*
    c. Local dull ache.
    d. Facial paralysis, mandibular pain.
15. Inframastoid (Imei I-ming) Figure 43.
    a. One fingerbreadth behind posterior earlobe below mastoid processus.

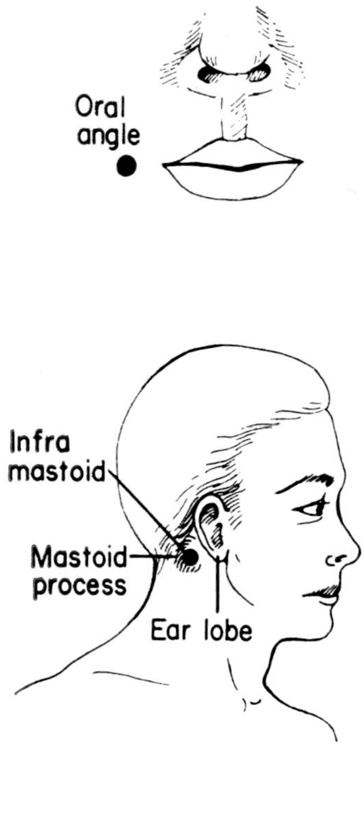

Figure 43: Lateral oral angle, inframastoid.

b. Pressure pain radiate to behind the ear and lateral neck.
c. Direct or oblique stick anteriorly for one inch.
d. Blindness.
e. Caution: potential danger to main trunk of facial nerve.

16. High lateral trapezius (Fuchi, fengs-chi) Figures 44 a and b.
    a. Groove lateral to the trapezius muscle and just above the hairline.
    b. Oblique stick one inch aiming opposite orbit.
    c. Radiate pressure pain to occipital or eye region.
    d. Migraine, dizziness, blindness, tinnitus.

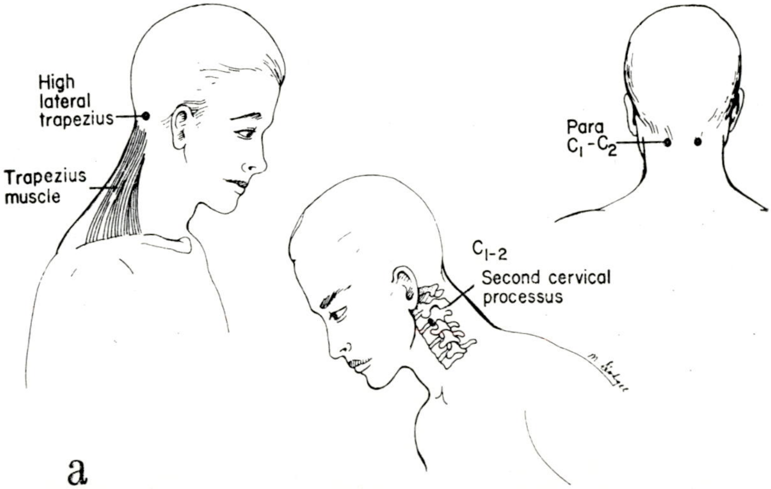

a

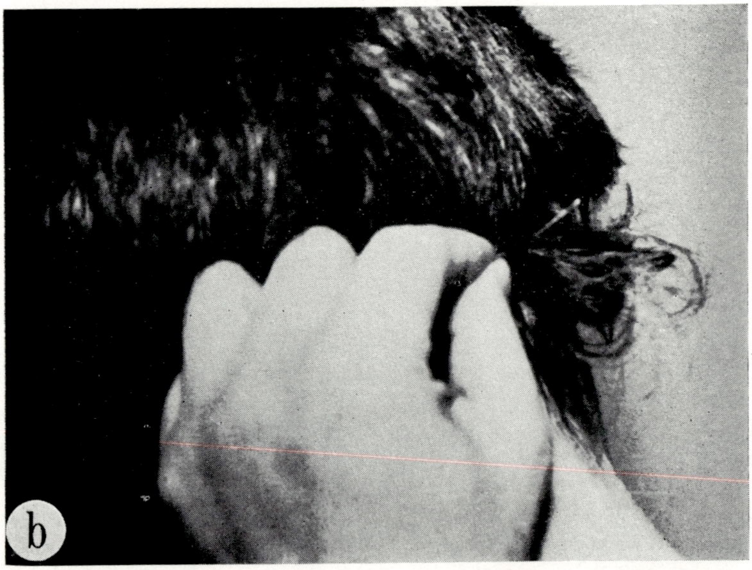

Figure 44: High lateral trapezius, C_1-C_2 (a) drawing, (b) photograph.

17. C1-C2 (Amon, ya-men) Figure 44a.
    a. Between the first and second cervical vertebrae one fingerbreadth above hairline at the posterior midline.
    b. Have the patient flex his neck and insert perpendicular stick one inch just above the second spinal process aiming toward the pharynx.
    c. When the needle reaches the ligament, resistance will be felt. Advance needle slowly and stop.
    d. Hypertension, mutism, pharyngitis, goiter.
18. Para C1-C2 (Tenchyu, Tien-chu) Figure 44a.
    a. Half fingerbreadth lateral of C1-C2 (lateral of trapezius muscle).
    b. Direct stick one inch aiming toward the opposite orbit.
    c. Radiate pain entire occipital area and eye. Immediate response with clear head and clear vision.
    d. Headache, insomnia, eye and nose diseases, hypertension, trigeminal neuraglia, shoulder pain.
19. Lateral thryoid (Jingei, Jen-ying) Figure 45.
    a. Extend neck, intersection of an imaginary line at the level of cricoid cartilage and anterior border of sternocleidomastoid muscle.
    b. Perpendicular stick one inch over pulsation of carotid artery.
    c. Paralyzing feeling to shoulder and elbow.
    d. Hypertension, mutism, pharyngitis, goiter.
20. Supra Sternum (Tentotsu, t'ien-t'u) Figures 46 and 47.
    a. Extend neck just above sternal notch behind sternum and front of trachea.
    b. Oblique stick one inch.

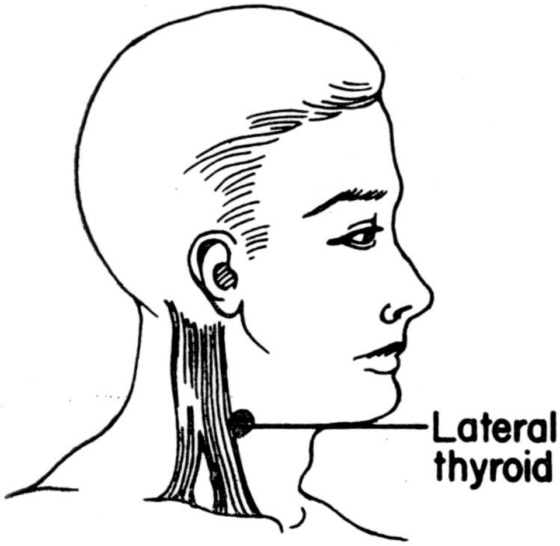

Figure 45: Lateral thyroid.

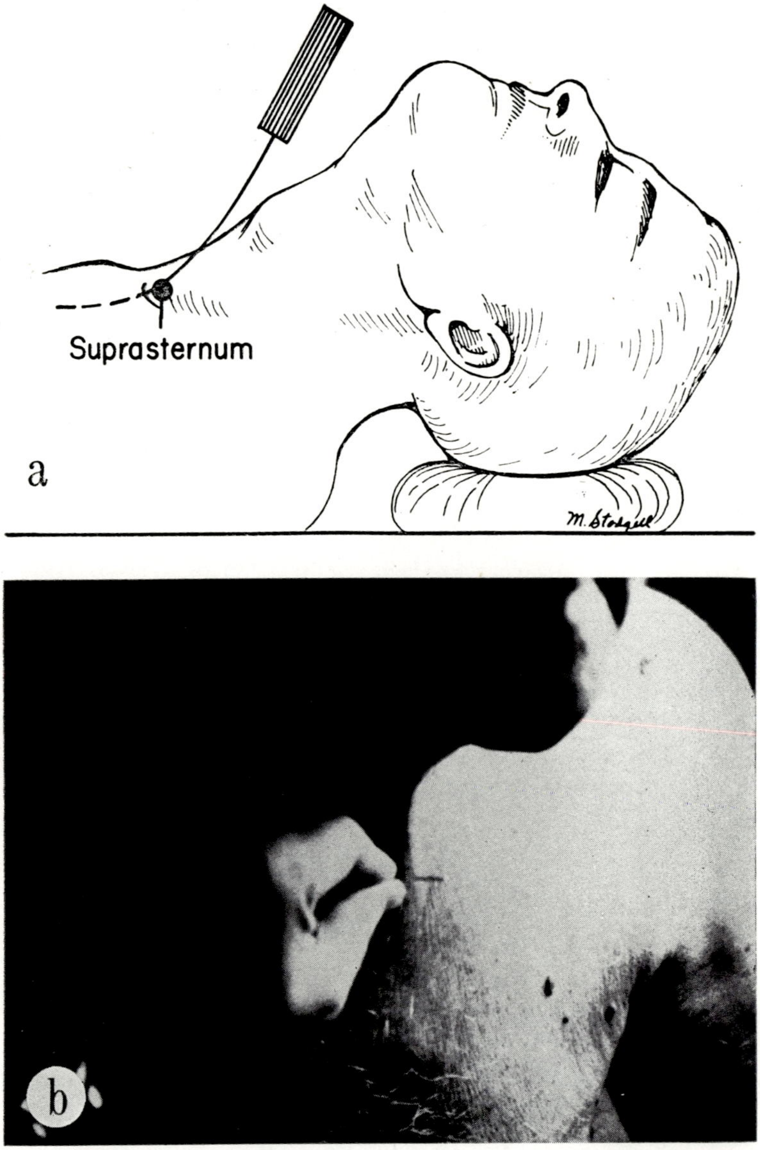

Figure 46: Suprasternum (a) drawing, (b) photograph.

c. Post sternal discomfort.
d. Dyspnea, mutism, vomiting, hiccups, pharyngitis.

21. C7-T1 (Daizui, ta-ch'ui) Figure 47.
  a. Flex head just below C7 which is the most prominent processus.
  b. Oblique stick one inch slightly upward.
  c. Paralyzing and pressure feeling in head, shoulders.
  d. Cold, back pain, fever, sprain, epilepsy.

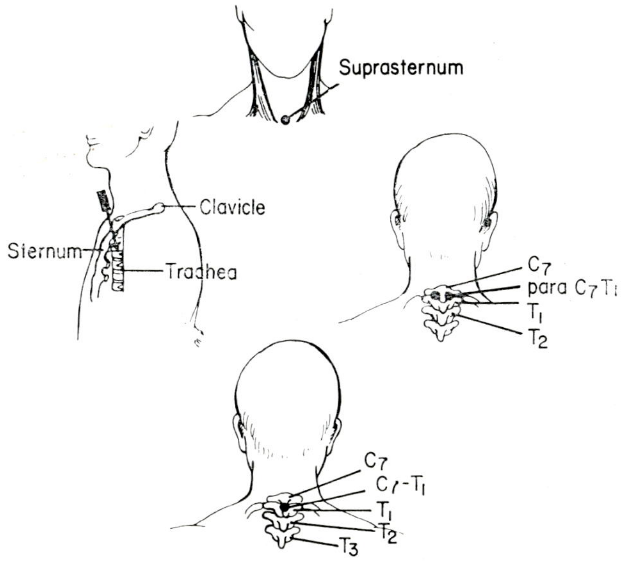

Figure 47: Suprasternum, C7—T1, Para C7—T1.

22. Para C7-T1 (Chizen) Figure 47.
    a. Lateral boney edge between C7 and T1.
    b. Perpendicular stick for one inch.
    c. Paralyzing or pressure feeling down to back.
    d. Asthma, cough, headache.
    e. Caution: Must be close to vertebrae, otherwise causes pneumothorax.

Chest and Abdomen

1. Midsternum (Danchyu, shan-chung) Figure 48.
    a. Fourth intercostal line at midsternum.

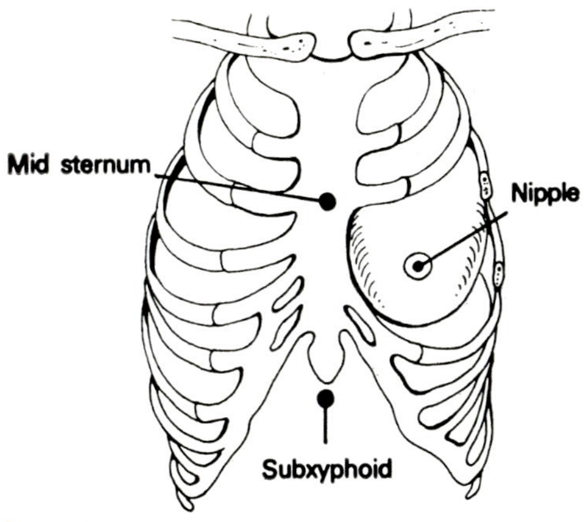

Figure 48: Midsternum, subxyphoid.

b. Subcutaneous stick for one inch.
c. Radiate to chest.
d. Asthma, URI, neurosis, heart disease.

2. Subxyphoid (kyubi, chiu-wei) Figure 48.
    a. Just below xyphoid process.
    b. Oblique stick one inch caudally.
    c. Psychosis, angina.
3. Sub-breast (Nyukon, Ju-keng) Figure 49.
    a. Base of breast at nipple line.
    b. Subcutaneous stick laterally.
    c. Local pressure.
    d. Mastitis.
4. Midepigastrium (Chyukan, chung-Wuan) Figure 49.
    a. Middle point between xyphoid and umbilicus.
    b. Perpendicular stick one inch, caution in hepatomegally.
    c. Paralyzing sensation of epigastrium.
    d. Abdominal pain, abdominal distentsion, diarrhea, meteorism, vomiting, constipation.

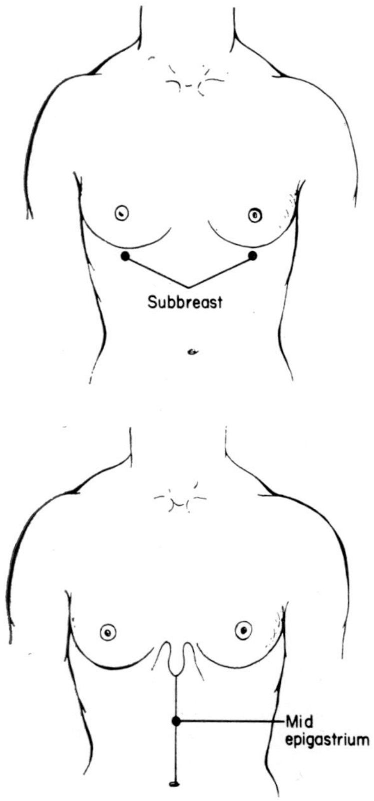

Figure 49: Sub-Breast, Midepigastrium.

5. Lateral Umbilicus (Tensu, t'ien-shu) Figure 50.
   a. Two fingerbreadth lateral from umbilicus.
   b. Perpendicular stick one inch.
   c. Paralyzing pressure sensation to lateral aspect of abdomen.
   d. Meteorism, diarrhea, abdominal pain, constipation, gynecological disorders.
6. Upper Hypogastrium (kikai, chi-hai) Figure 50.
   a. One-fifth distance below umbilicus to pubis.
   b. Direct stick one inch.
   c. Local pressure, occasional radiation to umbilicus.
   d. Abdominal pain.
7. Low Hypogastrium (Kangen, kuan-yuan) Figure 50.
   a. Three-fifth distance below umbilicus to pubis.
   b. Perpendicular stick one inch.
   c. Paralyzing pressure sensation to glands, penis or urethra.
8. Lower Hypogastrium (Chyu kyoku, chung-chi) Figure 50.
   a. Four-fifth below from umbilicus to pubis.
   b. Direct stick one inch.
   c. Local pressure, occasional radiation to umbilicus.
   d. GYN disorders, impotence, GU disorders, lower abdominal pain.
   e. Low hypogastrium and lower hypogastrium have similar effects

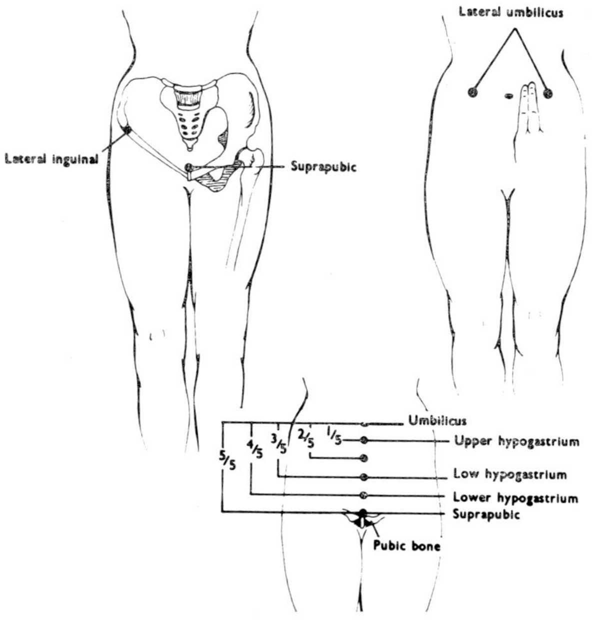

Figure 50: Lateral umbilicus, upper hypogastrium, low hypogastrium, lower hypogastrium, suprapubic, lateral inguinal.

but efficacy of low hypogastrium is a more systemic effect and that of lower hypogastrium is a more local effect.

9. Suprapubic (Kyoku kotsu, Chu-ku) Figure 50.
   a. Just above symphysis pubis.
   b. After voiding, direct stick one inch.
   c. Local pressure.
   d. Uterine prolapse.
10. Lateral Inguinal (Iho) Figure 50.
   a. One fingerbreadth median from superior anterior space of iliac bone.
   b. Oblique stick through inguinal canal two inches.
   c. Patient feels her uterus is ascending.
   d. Uterine prolapse.

Back

1. Para T2-T3 (Fumon, feng-men) Figure 51a.
   a. One and a half fingerbreadth lateral of midline between T2 and T3.
   b. Oblique stick half inch depth caudally.
   c. Radiate back and chest.
   d. Pneumonia, bronchitis, asthma, pleuritis, backache.
2. Para T3-T4 (Haiyu, feiyu) Lung Figure 51a.
   a. One and a half fingerbreadth lateral of midline between T2 and T3.
   b. Oblique stick caudally half inch depth.
   c. Radiate to back and chest.
   d. Cough, asthma, dyspnea, and respiratory disorders.

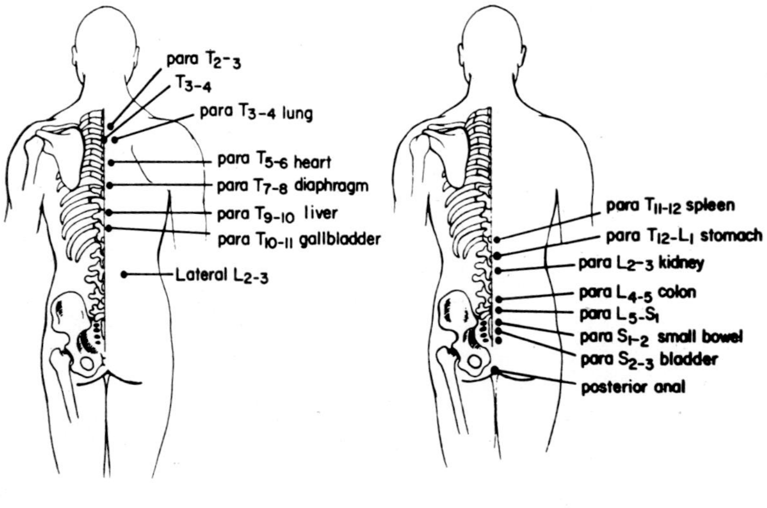

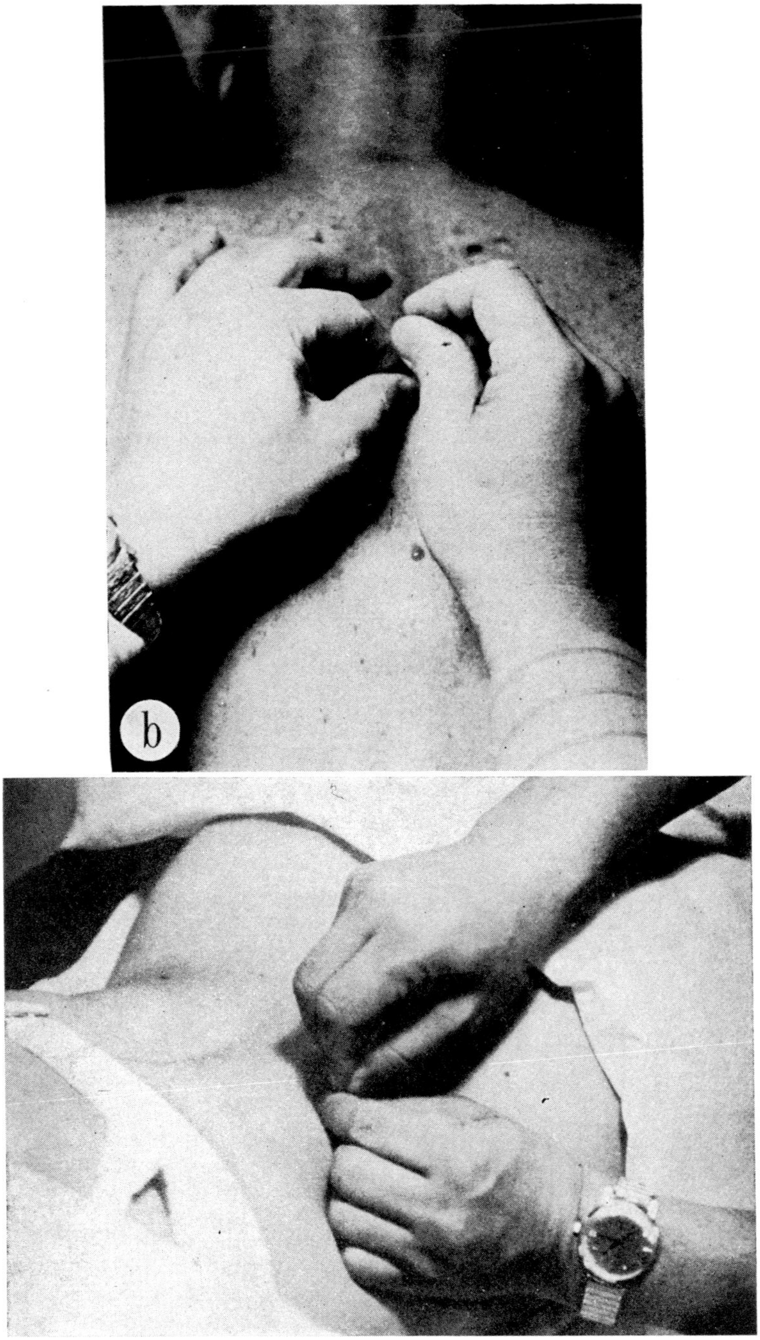

Figure 51: Para T2—T3; Para T3—T4; Para T5—T6; Para T7—T8; Para T9—T10; Para T10—T11; Para T11—T12; Para T12—L1; Para L2—L3; Para L3—L4; Para L4—L5; Para L5—S1; Para S1—S2; Lateral L2—L3; T3—T4; Posterior anal. (a) Drawing (b) Photograph—Para T5—T6 (c) Photograph—Lateral L2—L3.

3. Para T5-T6 (Shinyu, hsin-yu) Heart Figures 51 a and b.
   a. One and a half fingerbreadth lateral at midline between T5 and T6.
   b. Oblique stick caudally half inch depth.
   c. Back to chest.
   d. Tachycardia, heart diseases, cardiac asthma.
4. Para T7-T8 (Kakuyu, ke-yu) Diaphragm Figure 51a.
   a. One and a half fingerbreadth lateral of midline between T7 and T8.
   b. Oblique stick caudally half inch depth.
   c. Back to epigastrium.
   d. Asthma, pleuritis, gastritis—very important for treatment of chronic GI disorders.
5. Para T9-T10 Liver (Kanyu, Kenye) Figure 51a.
   a. One and a half fingerbreadth lateral of midline between T9 and T10.
   b. Oblique stick caudally half inch depth.
   c. Radiate back to epigastrium.
   d. Hepatitis, colic pain due to cholecystitis, gastric pain, backache, neurosis, liver and bilary diseases.
6. Para T10-T11 Gall Bladder (tanyu, tanyu) Figure 51a.
   a. One and half fingerbreadth lateral of midline between T10 and T11.
   b. Oblique stick half inch depth.
   c. Radiate to back.
   d. Diseases of biliary system, backache.
7. Para T11-T12 Spleen (Hiyu, p'i-yu) Figure 51a.
   a. One and a half fingerbreadth lateral of midline between T11 and T12.
   a. Oblique stick half inch depth.
   c. Radiate to back and umbilicus.
   d. Gastrointestinal disorders, peptic ulcer, pancreatitis, colitis enteritis, diabetes, joint rheumatism.
8. Para T12-L1 Stomach (Iyu, wei-yu) Figure 51a.
   a. One and a half fingerbreadth lateral of midline between T12 and L1.
   b. Oblique stick half inch depth.
   c. Radiate to back.
   d. Gastric disorders, backache, anoxia.
9. Para L2-L3 Kidney (jinyu, shen-yu) Figure 51a.
   a. Imaginary line between anterior superior iliac crest pass on L4.

b. One vertebra above that is L3.
c. One and a half fingerbreadth lateral of midline between L2 and L3.
d. Backache.
e. Caution: Danger of penetration of lumbar sac and cauda equina.

10 Para L4-L5 Colon (daichyoyu, ta-chang-yu) Figure 51a.
a. One and a half fingerbreadth lateral of midline between L4 and L5.
b. Oblique stick half inch depth.
c. Radiate to back.
d. Lumbosacral sprain sciatica, hip pain, colon diseases.

11. Para L5-S1 (Kangen-yu, Kuan-yuan-yu) Figure 51a.
a. One and a half fingerbreadth lateral of midline between L5 and S1.
b. Perpendicular stick one inch.
c. Radiate to gluteal or knee.
d. Dysmenorrhea, backache.

12. Para S1-S2 Small Bowel (shyochyoyu, hsiao-ch'ang-yu) Figure 51a.
a. One and a half fingerbreadth lateral of midline between S1 and S2.
b. Oblique stick half inch depth.
c. Radiate to back and gluteal area.
d. Low backache, hip pain, and intestinal diseases.

13. Para S2-S3 Bladder (bokoyu, p'ang-k'uang-yu) Figure 51a.
a. One and a half fingerbreadth lateral of midline between S2 and S3.
b. Oblique stick half inch depth.
c. Radiate to back and gluteal area.
d. Urinary disorders.

14. Lateral L2-L3 (shishitsu, chih-shih) Figures 51a and c.
a. Three fingerbreadths lateral of midline between L2 and L3; 1.5 fingerbreadth lateral of para L2-L3 (kidney point).
b. Perpendicular stick aiming medially two inches.
c. Radiate to entire back.
d. Specific for backache, renal diseases and impotence.

15. T3-T4 (mumec) Figure 51a.
a. Between T3 and T4.
b. Oblique stick half inch depth.
c. Radiate to back and shoulder.
d. Neurosis, hysteria, pediatric diseases, insomnia.

16. Posterior Anal (chyokyo, ch'ang-ch'iang) Figure 51a.

a. Midline between anus and coccyx.
b. Perpendicular superiorly for one inch.
c. Radiate anus and gluteal area.
d. Hemorrhoids, rectal diseases.

Upper Extremities

1. First Dorsal Metacarpal (Gokoku, ho-ku) Figures 52 a and b.

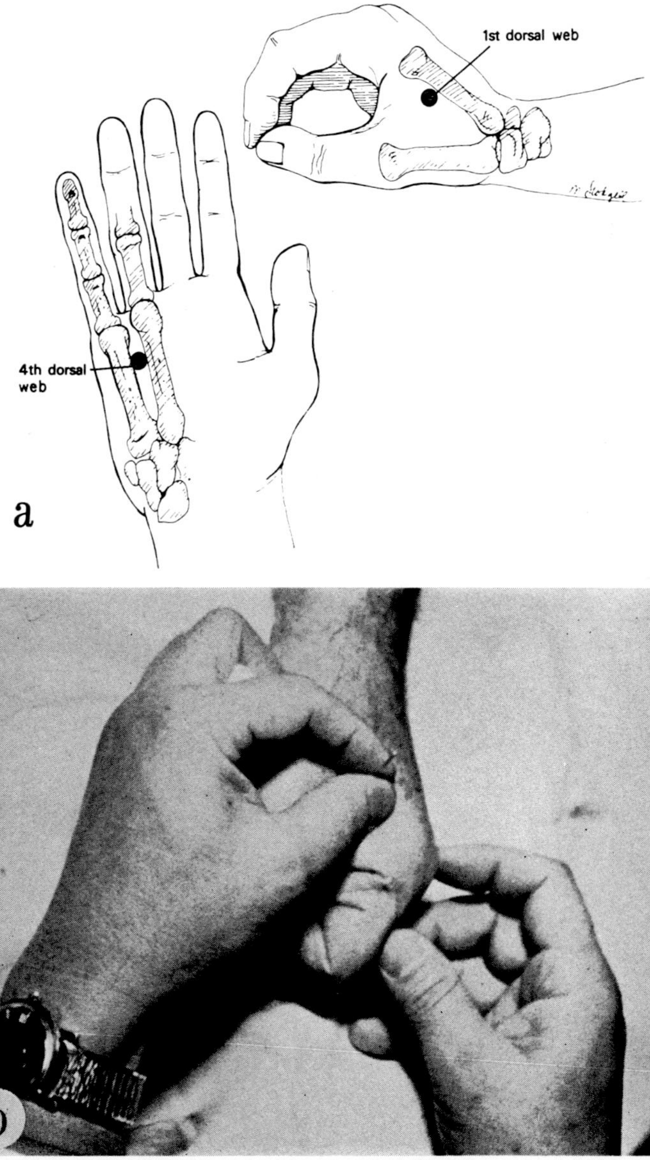

Figure 52: First dorsal web, fourth dorsal web, (a) drawing, (b) photograph.

a. The proximal point of the crease between first and second metacarpal space (the thumb and index finger).
b. Perpendicular stick one inch aiming fifth metacarpal.
c. Local pain, paralysis pressure to finger and shoulder.
d. Dental pain, tonsilitis, deafness, muteness, headache, rhinitis, eye diseases, anal pain, convulsion.
e. Contraindications for pregnant women.

2. Fourth Dorsal Metacarpal (Chyushyo, chung-chu) Figure 52a.
   a. Between fourth and fifth metacarpal bone at the dorsal aspect.
   b. Perpendicular stick half inch.
   c. Paralying sensation to fourth and fifth finger or shoulder.
   d. Deafness, tinnitis, pain at fourth and fifth fingers, shoulder pain.
3. Fifth Lateral Metacarpal (Kokei, hou-chi) Figure 53.
   a. Close hand and make a fist. Terminal point of major palmar crease.
   b. Perpendicular stick one inch.
   c. Aching on palmer aspect of hand.
   d. Do not repeat when painful.
   e. Neckache, backache, headache, deafness, tremor on face.
4. Dorsal Distal Forearm (Gaikan, wai-kuan) Figure 53.
   a. Two fingerbreadths from wrist crease between ulnar and radius.
   b. Perpendicular stick one inch.

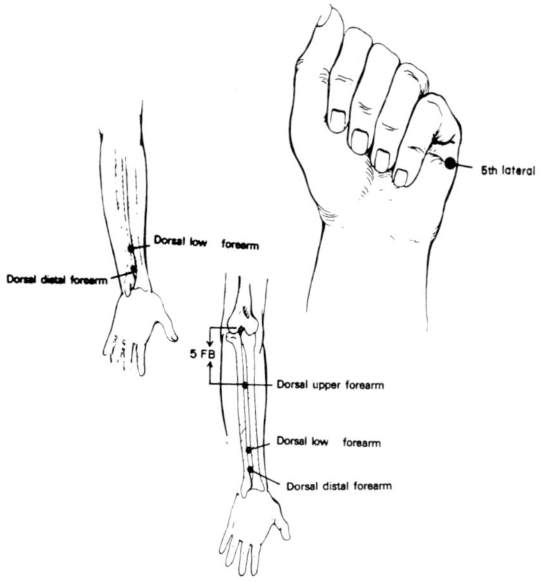

Figure 53: Fifth lateral metacarpal, dorsal distal forearm.

   c. Paralyzing and aching feeling or radiating sensation to third and fourth finger to shoulder.
   d. Wrist joint pain, migraine, deafness, elbow pain, upper arm paralysis.

5. Dorsal Low Forearm (Shiko, chih-kou) Figure 53.
   a. One fingerbreadth proximal of dorsal distal forearm.
   b. Perpendicular stick one inch.
   c. Paralyzing, pressure sensation to finger or upper arm.
   d. Habitual constipation.
6. Dorsal Upper Forearm (Shitoku, szu-tu) Figure 53.
   a. Five fingerbreadths distal from cubital crease at dorsal aspect.
   b. Perpendicular stick one inch.
   c. Paralyzing or radiating sensation to upper arm or down to hand.
   d. Migraine, forearm pain.
7. Radial Styloid Processus (Letsuketsu, lieh-ch'ueh) Figure 54.
   a. Styloid process of the radius.
   b. Oblique stick one inch aiming at elbow.
   c. Paralyzing and pressure sensation to elbow.
   d. Wrist joint pain, cough, headache.
8. Lateral cubital crease (Kyokuchi, chu-chih) Figure 54.
   a. Flex elbow 60° and lateral end of distal cubital crease.
   b. Perpendicular stick one inch deep.
   c. Paralyzing, radiating sensation to hand or shoulder.
   d. Hypertension, eczema, skin disease, shoulder pain, arm pain, hemiplegia, tonsilitis.

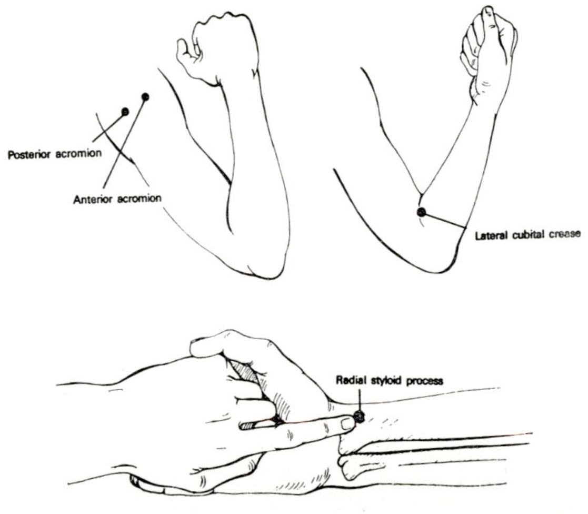

Figure 54: Posterior acromion, anterior acromion, lateral cubital crease, radial styloid process.

9. Volar Distal Forearm (Naikan, nei-kuan) Figure 55.
   a. Two fingerbreadths proximal from wrist crease between two central tendons.
   b. Perpendicular stick one inch.
   c. Paralyzing or pressure feeling to finger and shoulder.
   d. Upper abdominal pain, nausea, vomiting, hematemesis, chest pain, deafness, muteness, psychosis, paralysis of upper extremities.
10. Inter M.P. Joint (hachija, pa-hsieh) Figure 55.
    a. Make a fist and between each knuckle.
    b. Perpendicular stick 0.5 inch.
    c. Needle sensation along the finger.
    d. Pain and numbness of fingers and finger joints.
11. Finger Tip (Jissen, shih-hsuan) Figure 56.
    a. Finger tip.
    b. Blood letting or perpendicular stick.
    c. Sharp needle sensation locally.
    d. High fever, shock, paralysis of extremities.

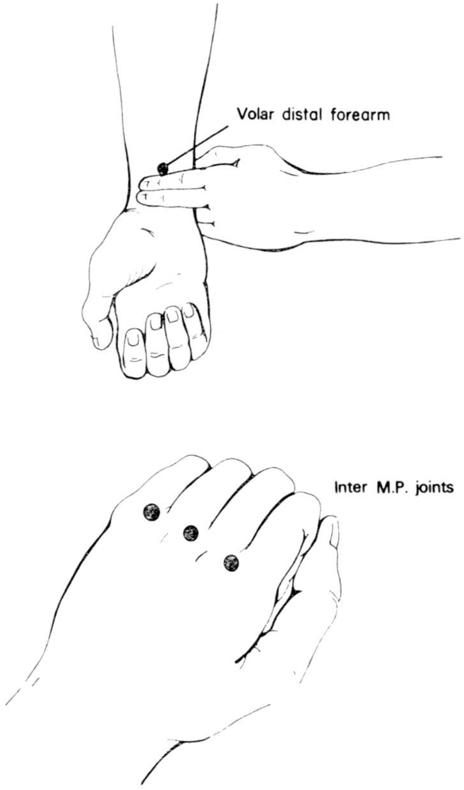

Figure 55: Volar distal forearm, inter M.P. joints.

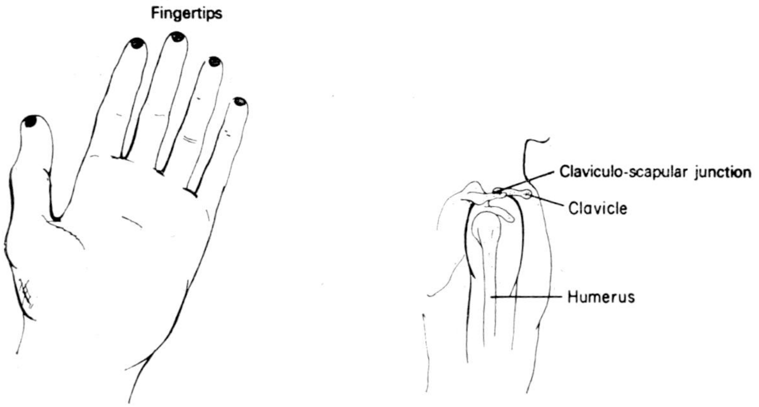

Figure 56: Fingertips, claviculo-scapular junction.

12. Claviculoscapular Junction (Kyokotsu, chu-ku) Figure 56.
    a. Depression between clavicle and scapua.
    b. Perpendicular stick one inch parallel to clavicle.
    c. Radiate to shoulder joint.
    d. Shoulder ache, shoulder joint pain, dental pain (lower jaw).
13. Anterior Acromion (Kengu, chien-yu) Figures 54, 57 a and b.
    a. Keep arm horizontal position immediately front of acromion.
    b. Perpendicular stick aiming clavicle for one inch.
    c. Dull ache radiating proximally and distally.
    d. Shoulder pain.
14. Posterior Acromion (Kenko, chien-liao) Figure 54.
    a. Keep arm horizontal position & immediately posterior to acromion.
    b. Perpendicular stick aiming axilla for one inch.
    c. Dull ache radiating proximally and distally.
    d. Shoulder pain, upper arm pain and paraylsis of upper arm.
15. Posterior axillary crease (Kentei, chien-chen) Figure 57.
    a. End point of posterior axillary fold.
    b. Perpendicular stick 1.0 inch.
    c. Dull ache to upper arm.
    d. Shoulder and upper arm pain, paralysis of upper arm.
16. Midlateral humerus (pi-nao) Figure 57.
    b. Perpendicular stick one inch
    c. Dull local ache radiating proximally and distally.
    d. Shoulder and upper arm pain.

Lower Extremities

1. Posterior trochanter (Kanchyo, huan-tiao) Figure 58.
    a. Two-thirds of distance of midline to trochanter on an imaginary line from greater trochanter of femur to coccyx.

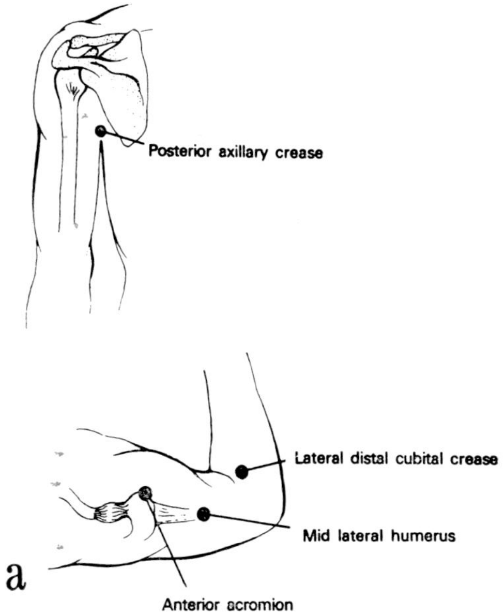

Figure 57: Posterior axillary crease, lateral distal cubital crease, mid-lateral humerus, anterior acromion, (a) drawing, (b) photograph.

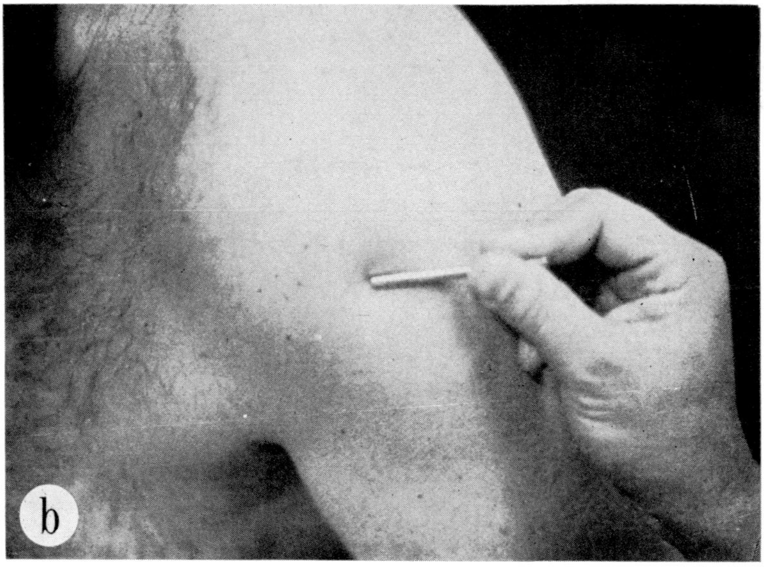

b. Aim for meridian inferior aspect for two inches.
c. Radiate to foot.
d. Back and thigh pain, hemiplegia, paralysis.

2. Midgluteal crease (Shiyofu, ch'eng-fu) Figures 58 a and b.
   a. Midline on the gluteal fold.
   b. Perpendicular stick two inches.
   c. Needle shock along leg to foot.

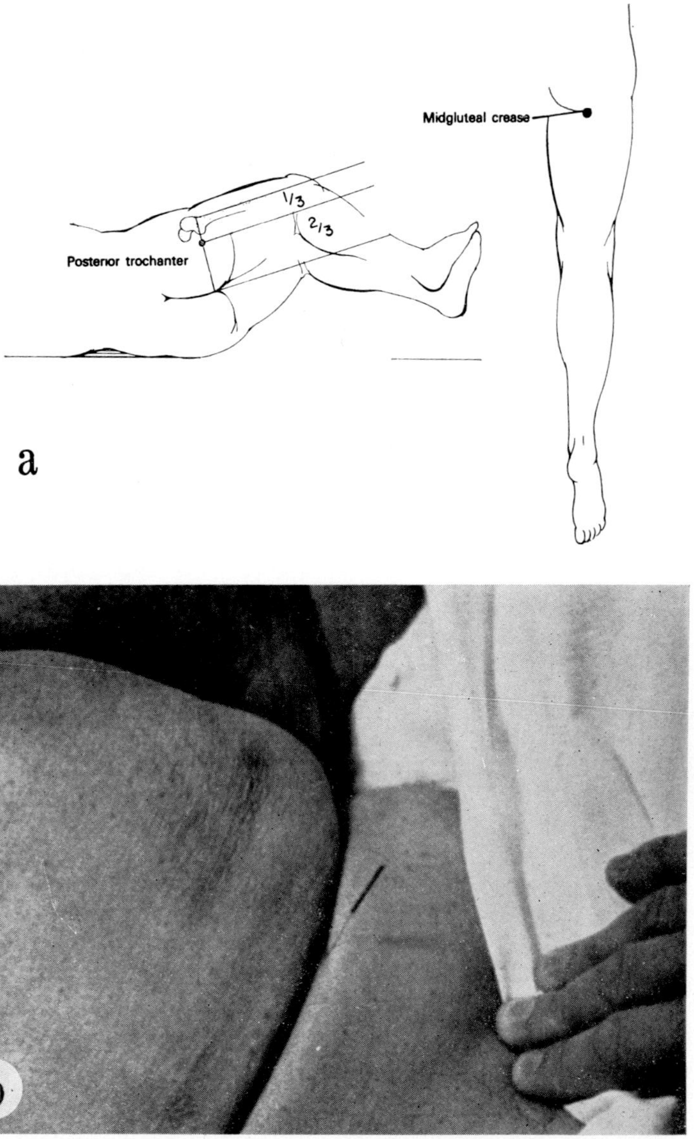

Figure 58: Posterior trochanter, midgluteal crease, (a) drawing, (b) photograph.

d. Sciatica, paralysis of lower extremities, hemorrhoids, urinary retention, backache.

3. Posterior midthigh (Yin mon, yin-men) Figure 59.
   a. Between gluteal crease and popliteal crease at midline.
   b. Perpendicular stick one inch.
   c. Radiating sensation.
   d. Pain in leg joint, pain and paralysis in lower extremities.

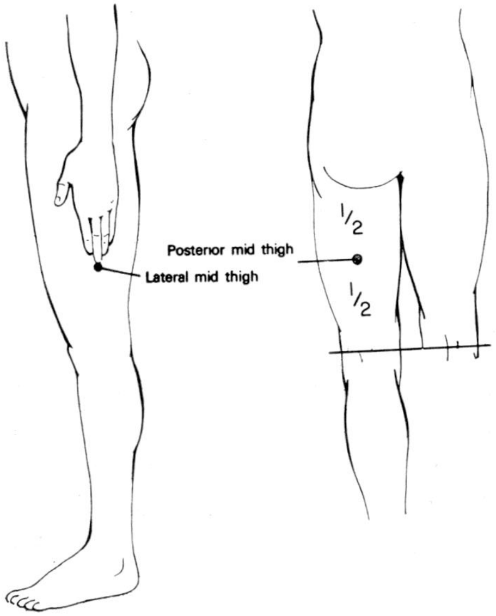

Figure 59: Posterior mid-thigh, lateral mid-thigh.

4. Lateral midthigh (Fuichi, fong-chih) Figure 59.
   a. In standing position with his arm hanging at his side, this point corresponds to tip of middle finger.
   b. Perpendicular stick two inches.
   c. Needle shock along leg to foot.
   d. Paralysis, lower extremities, back pain, neurodermatitis.
5. Lateral Upper Tibia (Ashi sanri, tsu-san-li) Figures 60 a and c.
   a. Three fingerbreadth inferior to lateral tibial tuberosity.

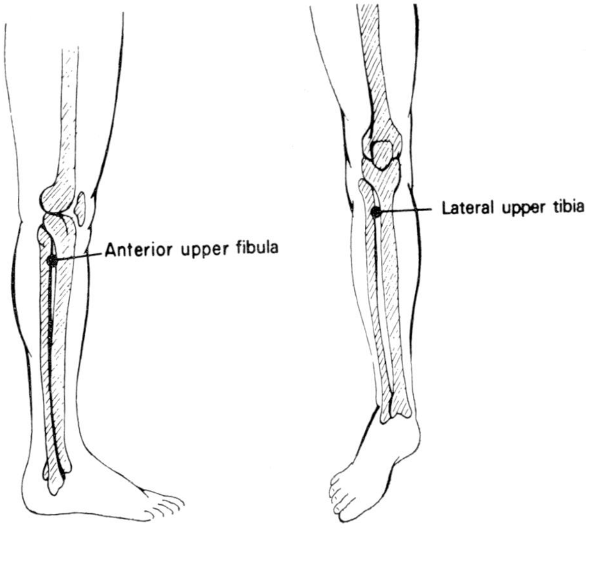

a

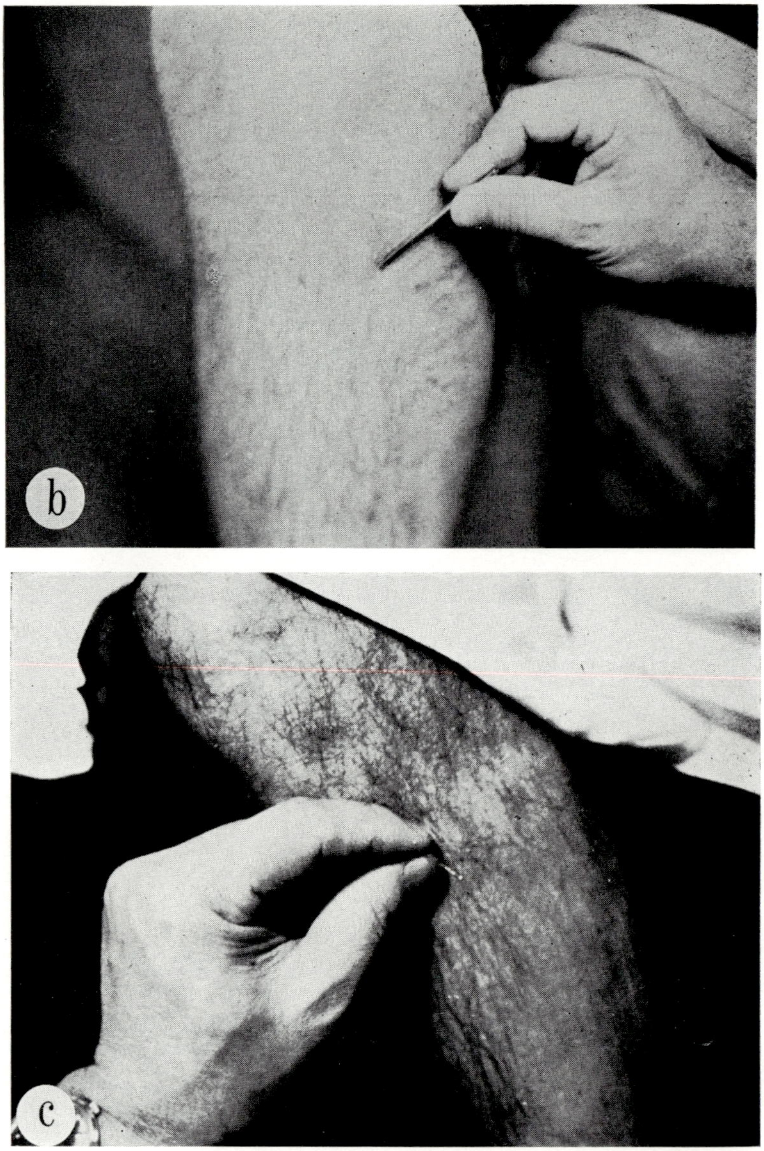

Figure 60: Anterior upper fibula, lateral upper tibia, (a) drawing, (b) photograph, (c) photograph.

b. Perpendicular stick one inch.
c. Radiation of paralyzing sensation to foot or perineum.
d. Dysuria, incontinency, urethral pain, impotence, hemiplegia, dysmenorrhea.

6. Anterior upper fibula (Yoryosen, yang-lin-chuan) Figures 60 a and b.
 a. Anterior to the neck of fibula.

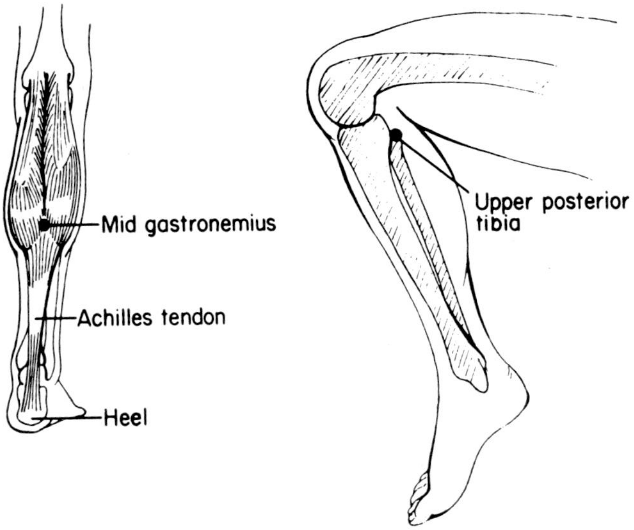

Figure 61: Mid-gastronemius, upper posterior tibia.

b. Perpendicular stick one inch.
c. Paralyzing or radiating sensation to foot or knee.
d. Knee pain, hemiplegia, lateral lower leg pain, bilateral chest pain.

7. Posterior upper tibia (Inryosen, yin-lin-ch'uan) Figures 61 and 65.
   a. Posterior to inferior portion of medialcondyl of tibia.
   b. Perpendicular stick one inch.
   c. Radiation or paralyzing sensation to foot or perineum.

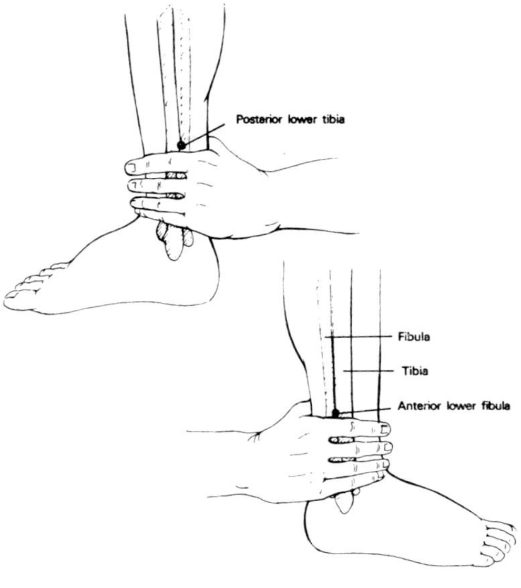

Figure 62: Posterior lower tibia, anterior lower fibula.

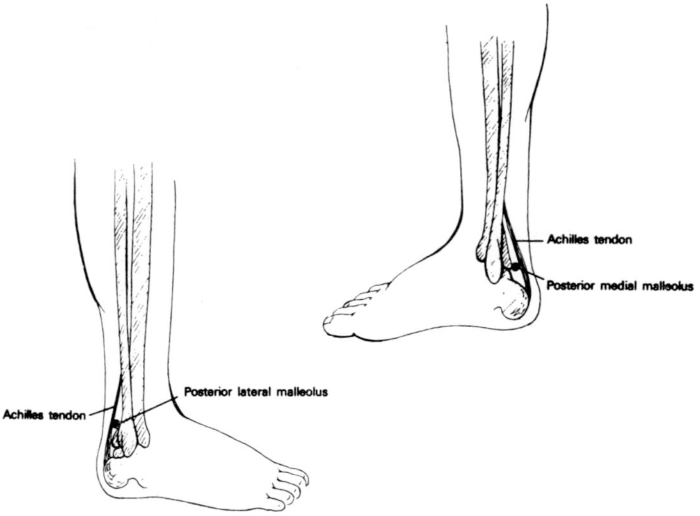

Figure 63: Posterior lateral malleolus, posterior medial malleolus.

d. Dysuria, incontinency, urethral pain, impotence, hemiplegia, dysmenorrhea.

8. Midgastrocnemius (Shyozan, ch'eng-san) Figure 61.
   a. Stand on toes, junction of medial and lateral heads of gastrocnemius muscle.
   b. Perpendicular stick two inches.
   c. Paralyzing pressure sensation to foot and knee.
   d. Calf pain.
9. Posterior Low Tibia (Saninko, san-yin-chiao) Figure 62.

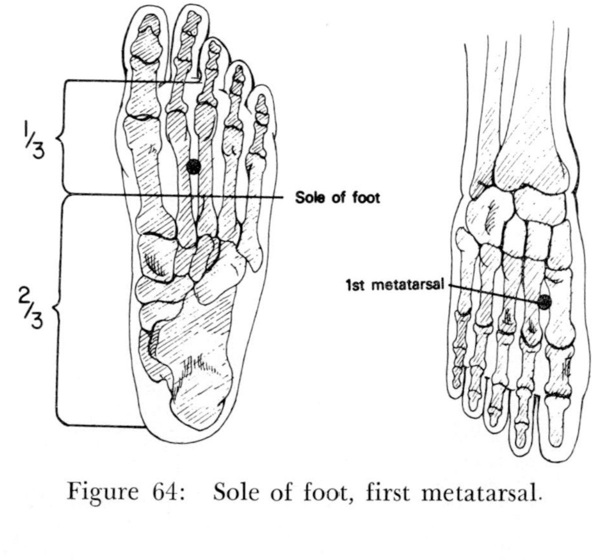

Figure 64: Sole of foot, first metatarsal.

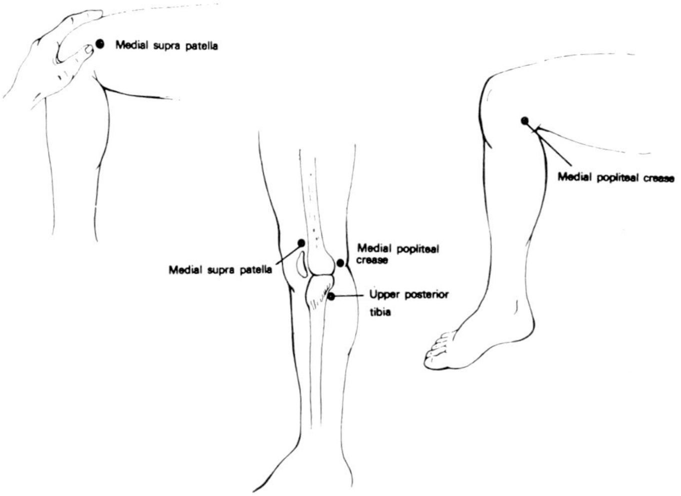

Figure 65: Medial supra patella, medial popliteal crease.

a. Four fingerbreadths proximal from medial malleolus of tibia at its posterior surface.
b. Perpendicular stick for one inch.
c. Paralyzing pressure sensation to sole of foot too tight.
d. Dysmenorrhea, impotence, insomnia, diabetes mellitus, GU problems.

10. Anterior lower Fibula (Zetsukotsu, chueh-ku) Figure 62.
    a. Four fingerbreadth proximal from lateral malleolus at its anterior surface.
    b. Perpendicular stick one inch.
    c. Paralyzing and radiating sensation to foot or even to shoulder.
    d. Foot joint pain, back and lower extremity pain, hemiplegia.
11. Posterior Lateral Malleolus (Konron, kun-chun) Figure 63.
    a. Between achilles tendon and lateral malleolus.
    b. Direct stick one inch.
    c. Paralyzing pressure sensation to foot or thigh.
    d. Foot joint pain, lower leg paralysis, backache, occipital headache, difficult OB problems.
12. Posterior Medial Malleolus (Taikei, tai-chi) Figure 63.
    a. Between achilles tendon and medial malleolus.
    b. Direct stick one inch.
    c. Paralyzing pressure sensation to foot.
    d. Foot joint pain, diabetes.
13. First intermetatarsal (Tai shiyo, t'ai-ch'ung) Figure 64.

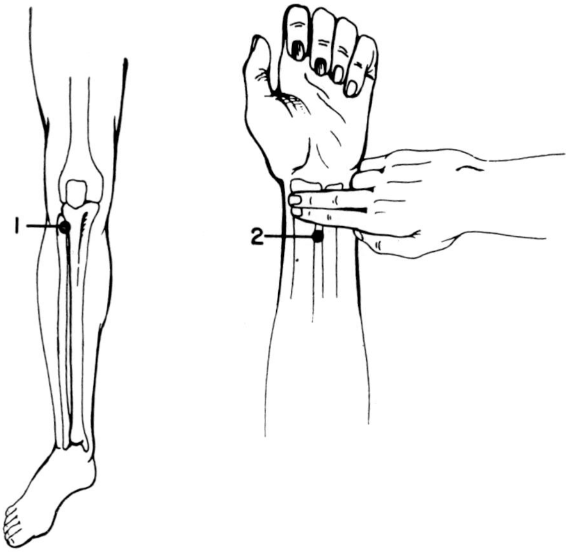

Figure 66: 1—Lateral upper tibia, 2—Volar distal forearm.

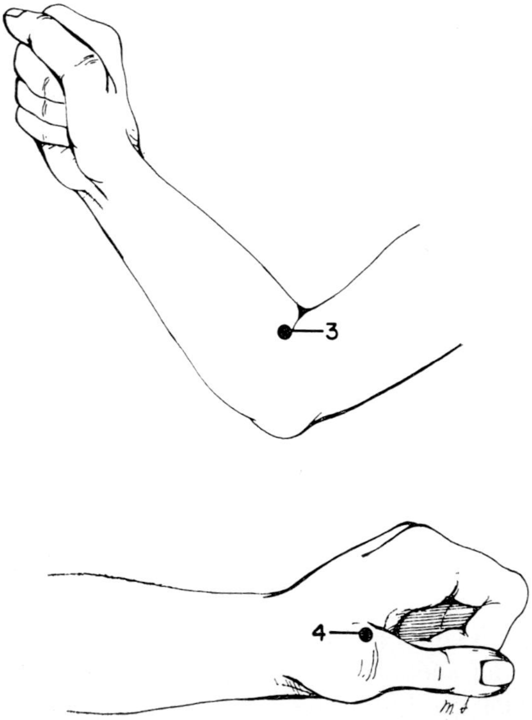

Figure 67: 3—Lateral cubital crease, 4—First dorsal web.

a. Two fingerbreadth proximal from dorsal aspect of junction between first and second toes.
b. Perpendicular stick one inch.
c. Paralyzing pressure sensation to toes or abdomen.
d. Headache, dizziness, throat pain.

14. Sole of Foot (Yosen, yung-ch'uan) Figure 64.
a. Two-thirds of distance from heel to base of toes at the midline of sole of foot.
b. Perpendicular stick one inch.
c. Tense pain at sole of foot.
d. Headache, unconsciousness.

15. Median Supra Patella (Ketsukai, hsueh-hai) Figure 65.
a. Two fingerbreadths above knee at median aspect of thigh.
b. Oblique stick, superficially two inches.
c. Local pressure.
d. Eczema, pruritus.

16. Median Popliteal Crease (Kyokusen, chu-chuan) Figure 65.
a. Median end of popliteal crease.
b. Perpendicular stick one inch.
c. Local pressure radiating pain to lower leg.
d. Nocturia, dysuria, impotence, knee pain.

This author attempted to choose a minimum number of the most commonly used and essential acupuncture points from over 360 meridian points and to create reasonable medical terminology for each of these.

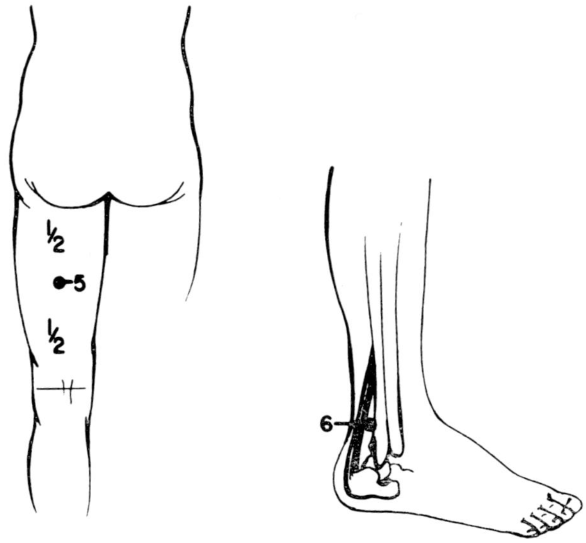

Figure 68: 5—Posterior mid-thigh, 6—Posterior lateral malleolus.

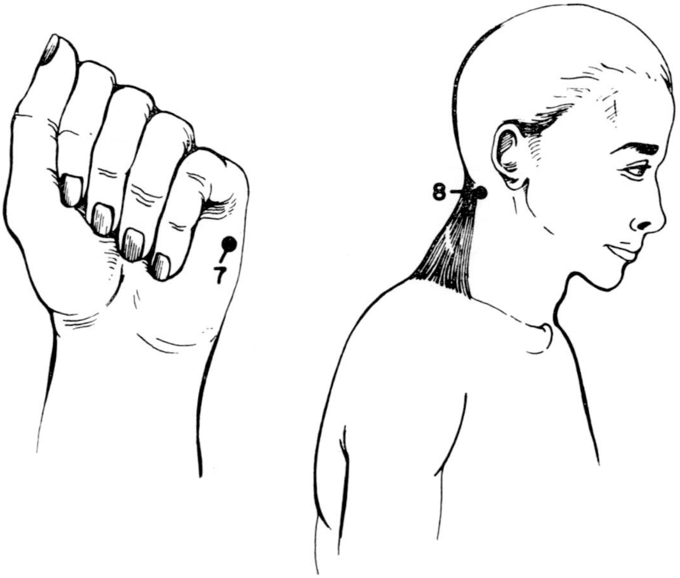

Figure 69: 7—Fifth lateral metacarpal, 8—High lateral trapezius.

The following ten points are the most commonly used and essential points and are considered as basic points.

1. Chest and Abdominal Diseases:
   a. Lateral upper tibia, (Ashi sanri: Tsu-san-li) Figure 66-1. Three fingerbreadths (FB) below tibial tuberosity.
   b. Volar distal forearm. (Naikwan: Nei-kuan) Figure 66-2. Two FB proximal to the wrist crease between the two central tendons.
2. Head and Face Ailments:
   a. Lateral cubital crease, (Kyokuchi: Chu-chih) Figure 67-3. Flex elbow 60° and find lateral end of distal cubital crease.
   b. First dorsal Web (Gokoku, Ho-ku) Figure 67-4. Adduct thumb tightly, find the point at the end of the crease.
3. Backache:
   a. Posterior Midthigh, (Inmon, Yin-men) Figure 68-5. Midpoint between gluteal and transverse popliteal folds on the posterior midline of the thigh.
   b. Posterior lateral malleolus, (Konron: Kun-lun) Figure 68-6. Point between the Achilles tendon and lateral malleolus.
4. Head and Neck Disorder:
   a. Fifth metacarpal, (ko Kei: Hou-ch'i) Figure 69-7. Make a fist and gently find a terminal point on the major palmar crease.
   b. High lateral trapezius, (Fuchi: Feng-chin) Figure 69-8. Groove lateral to the trapezius muscle and just above the hairline.

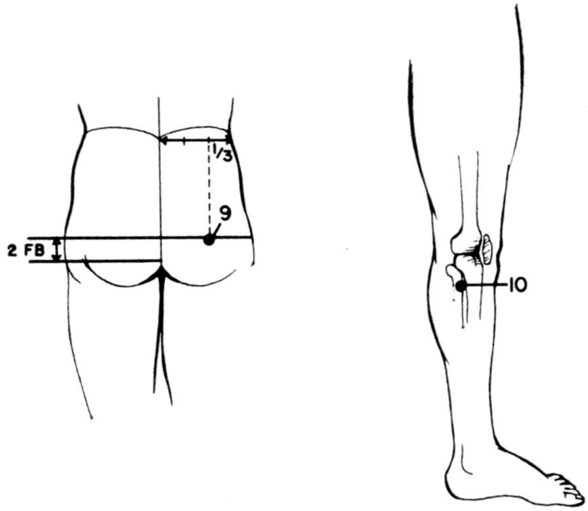

Figure 70: 9—Posterior trochanter, 10—Anterior upper fibula.

5. Knee, Chest and Side:
   a. Posterior Trochanter, (Kwanchiyo: Huan-tiao) Figure 70-9. Two-thirds lateral from the midline to the trochanter on an imaginary line between the greater trochanter of the femur and the coccyx.
   b. Anterior upper fibula, (Yoriyosen, Yang-lin-chuan) Figure 70-10. Immediately distal and anterior to the neck of the fibula.

SELECTION OF ACUPUNCTURE POINTS IN COMMON AILMENTS

I. ***Musculo-Skeletal Pain*** **(joint pain)**

A. *General*

1. Posterior Medial Malleolus (Taikei, Tai-chi) Figure 63.
   Posterior to medial malleolus and anterior to achilles tendon.
2. First Dorsal Web (Gokoku, Ho-ku) Figures 52 a and b.
   Radial volar aspect of the middle portion of the second metacarpal bone.
3. Fourth Dorsal Web (Chyu Chyo, Chung-chu) Figure 52.
   Between the fourth and fifth metacarpal bones and one finger-breadth proximal from the midpoint of the dorsum of the fourth metacarpal.
4. Vertex (Hyakue, Pe-hui) Figure 36.
   Midpoint of interaural line.

B. *Upper Extremities Including Shoulder Joint*

1. Radial Cubital Crease (Kyokuchi, Chu-chih) Figures 54 and 57.
   Flex elbow and point is at radial end of skin crease.
2. Dorsal Distal Forearm (Gaikan, Wai-kuan) Figure 53.

Two fingerbreadths proximal from dorsal wrist crease at midline.

3. First Dorsal Web (Gokoku, Ho-ku) Figures 52 a and b.
   Radia volar aspect of the middle portion of the second metacarpal bone.
4. Fifth Metacarpal (Kokei, Hou-chi) Figure 53.
   Make a fist and find ulnar end of transverse palmer crease.

C. *Lower Extremities*

1. Anterior Upper Fibula (Yoryosan, Yan-lin-chuan) Figures 60 a and b.
   One fingerbreadth below the anterior lateral aspect of fibular head.
2. Lateral Upper Tibia (Ashi-sanri, Tsu-san-li) Figures 60 a and c.
   Three fingerbreadths below tibial tuberosity and one fingerbreadth lateral of tibia.
3. Posterior Trochanter (Kachyo, Huan-tiao) Figure 58.
   Prone position, two fingerbreadths above upper end of transverse gluteal fold and two-thirds of distance of a line from midline to greater trochanter.

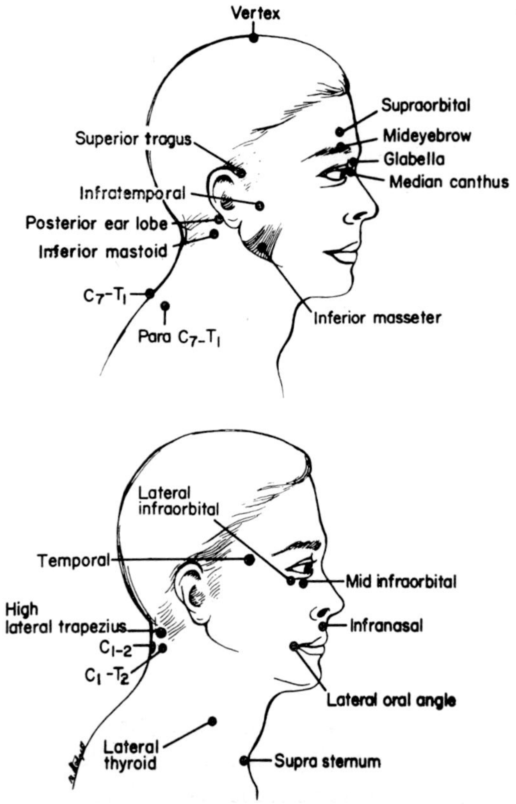

Figure 71: Related acupuncture points in head and neck.

4. Anterior Lower Fibula (Kenshyo) Figure 62.
   Four fingerbreadths above superior border of lateral malleolus and anterior border of fibula.

D. *Back Pain*

1. Post Mid-thigh (Inmon, Yin-men) Figure 59.
   At prone position, between middle of transverse gluteal fold and popliteal transverse crease.
2. Mid-gastrocnemius (Shyozan, Cheng-san) Figures 54 and 57.
   Stand on toes and find junction of two semicircular lines at inferior border of gastrocnemius muscle.
3. Posterior Lateral Malleolus (Konron, Kun-lun) Figure 63.
   Behind lateral malleolus and in front of Achilles tendon.
4. Fifth Metacarpal (Kokei, Hou-chi) Figure 53.
   Make a fist and find ulnar end of transverse palmer crease.
5. Para L2-L3 (Jinyu, Sheng-yu) Figure 51a.
   Prone position 1.5 fingerbreadths lateral of midpoint between spinous process of L2 and L3.
   Caution: Needle should be inserted carefully to avoid puncture of lumbar sac and cauda equina.

II. *Sprain*

A. *Neck*

1. Fifth Metacarpal (Kokei, Hou-chi) Figure 53.
   Make a fist and find ulnar end of palmer crease.
2. High Lateral Trapezius (Fuchi, Feng-chih) Figures 44 a and b.
   Between groove in trapezius muscle and mastoid process.

B. *Shoulder, Elbow, Arm*

1. Radial Cubital Crease (Kyokuchi, Chu-chih) Figures 54 and 57.
   Flex elbow and radial end of skin crease.
2. Dorsal Distal Forearm (Gaikan, Wai-kuan) Figure 53.
   Two fingerbreadths proximal from dorsal wrist crease at midline.

C. *Back*

1. Fifth Metacarpal (Kokei, Hou-chi) Figure 53.
   Make a fist and find ulnar end of palmer crease.
2. Posterior Upper Tibia (Inryosen, Yin-lin-chuan) Figures 61 and 65.
   At lower extremity, inferior. Posterior aspect of tibial head and just behind tibia.

D. *Hip*

1. Posterior Trochanter (Kanchyo, Huan-tiao) Figure 58.
   Prone position, two fingerbreadths above upper end of transverse gluteal fold and two-thirds of the distance of a line from midline to greater trochanter.

2. Anterior Lower Fibula (Kenshyo) Figure 62.
   Four fingerbreadths above superiod border of lateral malleolus and anterior border of fibula.

E. *Knee*

1. Anterior Upper Fibula (Yan-lin-chuan) Figures 60 a and b.
   One fingerbreadth below the anterior lateral aspect of fibular head.
2. Lateral Upper Tibia (Ashi sanri, Tsu-san-li) Figures 60 a and c.
   Three fingerbreadths below tibial tuberosity and one fingerbreadth lateral of anterior ridge of tibia.

F. *Ankle*

1. Posterior Lateral Malleolus (Konron, Kun-lun) Figure 63.
   Behind lateral malleolus and in front of Achilles tendon.
2. Anterior Lower Fibula (Kenshyo) Figure 62.
   Four fingerbreadths above superior border of lateral malleolus and anterior border of fibula.

III. *Dental Pain*

1. First Dorsal Web (Gokoku, Ho-ku) Figures 52 a and b.
   Radial volar aspect of the mid-portion of the second metacarpal bone.
2. Inferior Masseter (Kyoshiya, Chia-che) Figure 39.
   Between masseter muscle in front of mandibular angle at tight occlusion of teeth.
3. Infra Temporal (Gekan, Hsia-kuan) Figure 39.

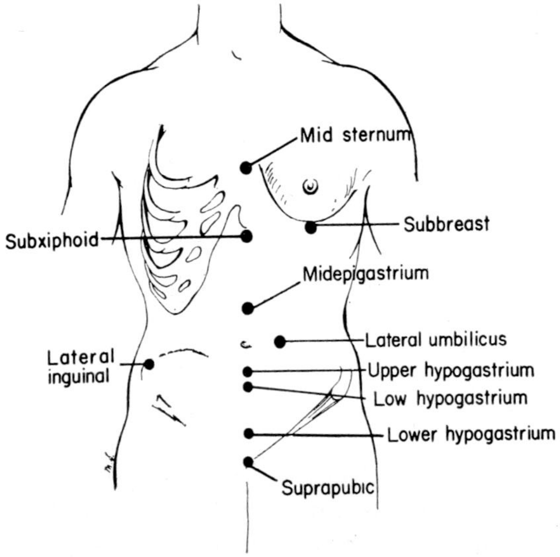

Figure 72: Related acupuncture points in chest and abdomen.

Infra zygomatic arch in front of tragus.
Caution: There are branches of facial nerve in this area.

IV. *Headache*

A. *Migraine*

1. Dorsal Distal Forearm (Gaikan, Wai-kian) Figure 53.
   Two fingerbreadths proximal from dorsal wrist crease.
2. Dorsal Upper Forearm (Shitoku) Figure 53.
   One-half the distance from wrist to elbow between radius and ulna.
3. High Lateral Trapezius (Fuchi, Feng-chih) Figures 44 a and b.
   Between trapezius muscle and mastoid process.
4. Temporal Fossa (Taiyo, Tai-yang) Figures 37 a and b.
   One fingerbreadth behind the midpoint between lateral end of eyebrow and eye.
   Caution: Small branch of facial nerve here. If damaged, patient might not be able to close eye.

B. *Entire Head*

1. Glabella (Indo, Yin-tang) Figure 38.
   Between two eyebrows, just above nasion.
2. C1-C2 (Amon, Ya-men) Figure 44a.
   Flex head, between C1 and C2 at midline.
   Caution: Be careful of depth of needle because the spinal cord can be penetrated.
3. Lateral Upper Tibia (Ashi sanri, Tsu-san-li) Figures 60 a and c.
   Three fingerbreadths below tibial tuberosity and one fingerbreadth lateral of anterior ridge of tibia.

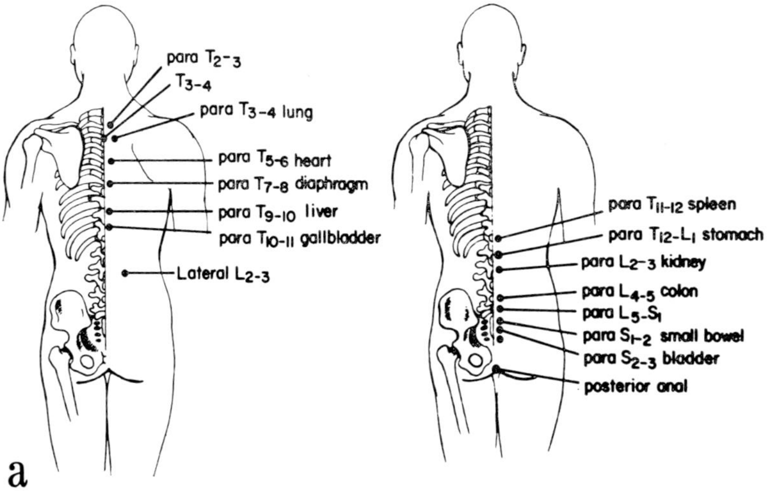

a

Figure 73: Related acupuncture points in back.

4. First Dorsal Metacarpal Web (Gokuku, Ho-ku) Figures 52 a and b. Radial volar aspect of the middle portion of the second metacarpal bone.
5. Dorsal Upper Forearm (Shitoku) Figure 53. One-half the distance from wrist to elbow between radius and ulna.
6. Temporal fossa (Taiyo, Tai-yang) Figures 37 a and b. One fingerbreadth behind the midpoint between lateral end of eyebrow and eye. (Caution about orbital branch of facial nerve).
7. T3-T4 (Shinchyu) Figure 51a. Below T3 process.
8. Para T5-T6 (Shinyu, Hsin-yu) Figures 51 a and b. Two fingerbreadths lateral of midline and below T5 process.

V. *Chest Pain*

1. Volar Distal Forearm (Naikan, Nei-kuan) Figure 55. Two fingerbreadths proximal from volar wrist crease at midline.
2. Anterior Upper Fibula (Yoryosen, Yau-lin-chuan) Figures 60 a and b. One fingerbreadth below the anterior lateral aspect of fibular head.
3. Midepigastrium (Chiyukan, chung-kuan) Figure 49. Midway between xyphoid and umbilicus.
4. Para T7-T8 (Kakuyu, Ke-yu) Figure 51a. Two fingerbreadths lateral below T7 spinous process.

VI. *Upper Abdominal Pain*

1. Volar Distal Forearm (Naikan, Nei-kuan) Figure 55. Two fingerbreadths proximal from volar wrist crease at midline.

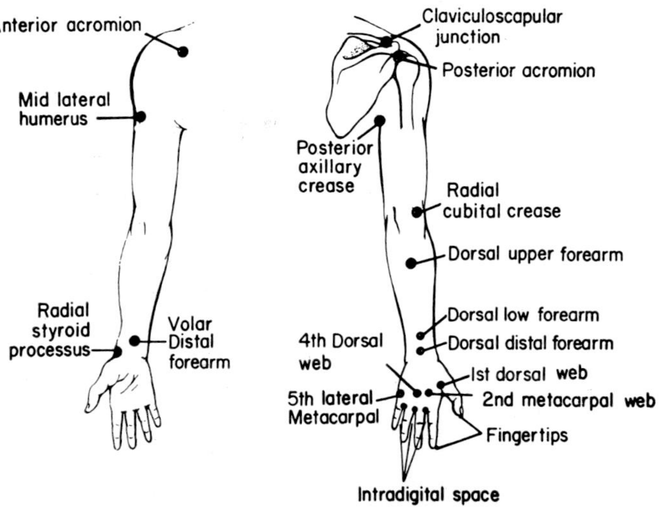

Figure 74: Related acupuncture points in upper extremeties.

2. Lateral Upper Tibia (Ashi sanri, Tsu-san-li) Figures 60 a and c.
Three fingerbreadths below tibial tuberosity and one fingerbreadth lateral of anterior ridge of tibia.
3. Posterior Low Tibia (Saninko, San-yin-chiao) Figure 62.
Four fingerbreadths above medial malleolus and behind tibia.
4. Posterior Upper Tibia (Inryosen, Yin-lin-chuan) Figures 61 and 65.
At median aspect of lower extremity, inferior and posterior to tibial head.
5. Midepigastrium (Chiyu kan, Chung-huan) Figure 49.
Between xyphoid and umbilicus.

VII. *Lower Abdominal Pain*

1. Low hypogastrium (Kangen, Kuan-yuan) Figure 50.
At midline three-fifths distance below umbilicus to pubis.

VIII. *Tonsilitis and Pharyngitis*

1. First Dorsal Web Metacarpal (Gokoku, Ho-ku) Figures 52 a and b.
Radial volar aspect of the middle portion of the second metacarpal bone.
2. Radial Cubital Crease (Koyokuchi, Chih) Figures 54 and 57.
Flex elbow and radial end of skin crease.
3. Supra Sternum (Tentotsu, Tien-tu) Figures 46 and 47.
Caution: Depth of needle and sterility are important because of danger of mediastinitis.

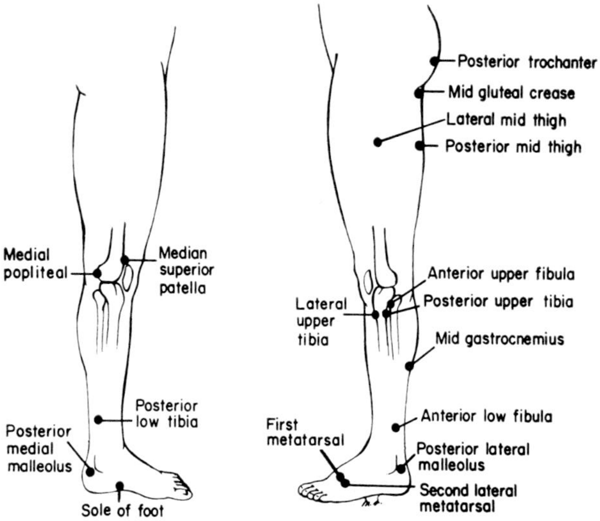

Figure 75: Related acupuncture points in lower extremeties.

4. Lateral Thyroid (Jingei) Figure 45.
   Extend neck, anterior border of sternocleidomastoid muscle at the level of the larynx.

IX. *Chronic Cough*

1. Suprasternum (Tentotsu, Tien-tu) Figures 46 and 47.
   Suprasternal notch.
   Caution: Depth of needle and sterility are important because of danger of mediastinitis.
2. Volar Distal Forearm (Naikan, Nei-kuan) Figure 55.
   Two fingerbreadths proximal from volar wrist crease at midline.
3. Lateral Upper Tibia (Ashi sanri, tsu-san-li) Figures 60 a and c.
   Three fingerbreadths below tibial tuberosity and one fingerbreadth lateral of tibia.
4. Para C7-T1 (Chizen) Figure 47.
   Two fingerbreadths lateral of the point between C7 and T1 spinous processes.

X. *Asthma*

1. Para C7-T1 (Chizen) Figure 47.
   Two fingerbreadths lateral of the point between C7 and T1.
2. Suprasternum (Tentotsu, Tien-tu) Figures 46 and 47.
   Suprasternal notch.
   Caution: Depth of needle and sterility are important because of danger of mediastinitis.
3. Lateral Upper Tibia (Ashi sanri, Tsu-san-li) Figures 60 a and c.
   Three fingerbreadths below tibial tuberosity and one fingerbreadth lateral of tibia.
4. First Dorsal Web (Gokoku, Ho-ku) Figures 52 a and b.
   Radial volar aspect of the middle portion of the second metacarpal bone.
5. Lateral Umbilicus (Tensu, Tein-shu) Figure 50.
   Two fingerbreadths lateral of umbilicus (right and left).
6. Para T-11-T-12 (Hiye, Pi-yu) Figure 51a.
   Two fingerbreadths lateral of below T11-T12.
7. Low hypogastrium (Kangen, Kuan-yuan) Figure 50.
   At midline on a line from pubis to umbilicus, three fingerbreadths below umbilicus.

XI. *Constipation*

1. Dorsal Low Forearm (Shiko) Figure 53.
   One fingerbreadth above gaikan (dorsal distal forearm).

2. Radial Cubital Crease (Kyukuchi, chu-chih) Figures 54 and 57.
   Flex elbow and radial end of skin crease.
3. First Dorsal Web (Gokoku, Hoku) Figures 52 a and b.
   Radial volar aspect of the middle portion of the second metacarpal bone.
4. Lateral Umbilicus (Tensu, Tien-shu) Figure 50.
   Two fingerbreadths lateral of umbilicus, both right and left.
5. Lateral Upper Tibia (Ashi-sanri, Tsu-san-li) Figures 60 a and c.
   Three fingerbreadths below tibial tuberosity and one fingerbreadth lateral of tibia.

XII. *Vomiting*

1. Volar Distal Forearm (Naikan, Nei-kuan) Figure 55.
   Two fingerbreadths proximal from volar wrist crease at midline.
2. Suprasternum (Tentotsu, Tien-tu) Figures 46 and 47.
   Suprasternal notch.
   Caution: Depth of needle and sterility are important because of danger of mediastinitis.
3. Lateral Upper Tibia (Ashi sanri, Tsu-san-li) Figures 60 a and c.
   Three fingerbreadths below tibial tuberosity and one fingerbreadth lateral of tibia.

XIII. *Gastric Atony*

1. Lateral Upper Tibia (Ashi sanri, Tsu-san-li) Figures 60 a and c.
   Three fingerbreadths below tibial tuberosity and one fingerbreadth lateral of tibia.
2. Para T12-L1 (Iyu wei-yu) Figure 51a.
   Two fingerbreadths lateral below T12.
3. Posterior Low Tibia (Saninko, Sanyin-chiao) Figure 62.
   Four fingerbreadths above medial malleolus and beind tibia.
4. Midepigastrium (Chiyukan, Chung-kuan) Figure 49.
   Midline between xyphoid and umbilicus.
5. Radial Cubital Crease (Kyokuchi, chu-chih) Figures 54 and 57.
   Flex elbow and radial end of skin crease.
6. First Dorsal Metacarpal Web (Gokoku, Ho-ku) Figures 52 a and b.
   Radial volar aspect of the middle portion of the second metacarpal bone.
7. Lateral Umbilicus (Tensu, Tien-shu) Figure 50.
   Two fingerbreadths lateral of umbilicus (both right and left).
8. Low hypogastrium (Kangen, Kuan-yuan) Figure 50.
   Three fingerbreadths below umbilicus at midline on a line from pubis to umbilicus.

9. Para T7-T8 (Kakuyu, Ke-yu) Figure 51a.
   Two fingerbreadths lateral below T7 spinous process.
10. Para L2-L3 (Kinyu, sheng-yu) Figure 51a.
    Prone position 1.5 fingerbreadths lateral of midpoint between spinous process of L2 and L3.
    Caution: Needle should be inserted carefully to avoid puncture of lumbar sac and cauda equina.
11. Posterior Lateral Malleolus (Konron, Kun-lun) Figure 63.
    Behind lateral malleolus and in front of Achilles tendon.

XIV. *Enuresis (Bed-wetting)*

1. Low hypogastrium (Kangen, kuan-yuan) Figure 50.
   At midline on a line from pubis to umbilicus, three fingerbreadths below umbilicus.
2. Posterior Low Tibia (Saninko, San-yiu-chiao) Figure 62.
   Four fingerbreadths above medial malleolus and behind tibia.
3. Lower hypogastrium (Chyukyoku, Chung-chi) Figure 50.
   Three fingerbreadths below umbilicus at midline on a line from pubis to umbilicus.
4. Lateral Upper Tibia (Ashi sanri, Tsu-san-li) Figures 60 a and c.
   Three fingerbreadths below tibial tuberosity and one fingerbreadth lateral of tibia.

XV. *Sleeplessness*

1. Lateral Upper Tibia (Ashi sanri, Tsu-san-li) Figures 60 a and c.
   Three fingerbreadths below tibial tuberosity and one fingerbreadth lateral of tibia.
2. Volar Distal Forearm (Naikan, Nei-kuan) Figure 55.
   Two fingerbreadths proximal from volar wrist crease at midline.
3. Posterior Low Tibia (Saninko, San-yin-chiao) Figure 62.
   Four fingerbreadths above medial malleolus and behind tibia.
4. High lateral Trapezius (Fuchi, Feng-chin) Figures 44 a and b.
   Between trapezius muscle and mastoid process.

XVI. *Hemiplegia*

1. Radial Cubital Crease (Kiyokuchi, chu-chih) Figures 54 and 57.
   Flex elbow and radial end of skin crease.
2. Anterior Upper Fibula (Yoriyosen, Yan-liu-chuan) Figures 60 a and b.
   One fingerbreadth below the anterior lateral aspect of the fibular head.
3. First Dorsal Metacarpal Web (Gokoku, ho-ku) Figures 52 a and b.
   Radial volar aspect of the middle portion of the second metacarpal bone.

4. Dorsal Distal Forearm (Gaikan, Wai-kuan) Figure 53.
   Two fingerbreadths proximal from dorsal wrist crease at midline.

XVII. *Anemia*

1. Lateral Upper Tibia (Ashi sanri, Tsu-san-li) Figures 60 a and c.
   Three fingerbreadths below tibial tuberosity and one fingerbreadth lateral of tibia.
2. Lateral Cubital Crease (Kiyokuchi, chu-chih) Figures 54 and 57.
   Flex elbow and radial end of skin crease.

XVIII. *Dysuria*

1. Lower Hypogastrium (Chyu kyoku, Chung-chi) Figure 50.
   At midline on a line from pubis to umbilicus, four-fifths distance below umbilicus.
2. Posterior Low Tibia (Saninko, San-yiu-chiao) Figure 62.
   Four fingerbreadths above medial malleolus and behind tibia.
3. Posterior Upper Tibia (Knryosen, Yin-lin-chuan) Figures 61 and 65.
   At median aspect of lower extremity, inferior and posterior to tibial head.

XIX. *Unconsciousness*

1. Infranasal (Kinchyu, jen-chung) Figure 42.
   One third of the distance of a line from anterior nasal spine to upper lip.
2. Volar Distal Forearm (Naikan, Nei-kuan) Figure 55.
   Two fingerbreadths proximal from volar wrist crease at midline.
3. Lateral Upper Tibia (Ashi sanri, Tsu-san-li) Figures 60 a and c.
   Three fingerbreadths below tibial tuberosity and one fingerbreadth lateral of tibia.

XX. *Convulsions*

1. First Dorsal Metacarpal Web (Gokoku, Ho-ku) Figures 52 a and b.
   Radial volar aspect of the middle portion of the second metacarpal bone.
2. Fifth Metacarpal (Kokei, Hou-chi) Figure 53.
   Make a fist and find ulnar end of palmar crease.
3. High Lateral Trapezius (Fuchi, feng-chih) Figures 44 a and b.
   Between trapezius muscle and mastoid process.

XXI. *Deafness*

1. C1-C2 (Amon, Ya-men) Figure 44a.
   Flex head, between C1 and C2 at midline.

Caution: Be careful of depth, can impale cord, cause paralysis, meningitis.

2. Suprasternum (Tentotsu, Tien-tu) Figures 46 and 47.
   Suprasternal notch (Depth of needle and sterility are important because of danger of mediastinitis).
3. Lateral Thyroid (Jingei) Figure 45.
   Extended neck, anterior border of sternocleidomastoid muscle at the level of the larynx.
4. Volar Distal Forearm (Naikan, Nei-kuan) Figure 55.
   Two fingerbreadths proximal from volar wrist crease at midline.
5. First Dorsal Web (Gokoku, Ho-ku) Figures 52 a and b.
   Radial volar aspect of the middle portion of the second metacarpal bone.
6. Fifth Dorsal Metcarpal (Kokei, Hon-chi) Figure 53.
   Make a fist and find ulnar end of palmar crease.

XXII. *Tinnitus*

1. Superior Tragus (Jimon, Erh-men) Figure 41.
   Immediately above tragus.
2. Posterior Earlobe and Mastoid. (fifu, I-feng) Figure 42.
3. Dorsal Distal Forearm (Gaikan, Wai-kuan) Figure 53.
   Two fingerbreadths proximal from dorsal wrist crease in midline.
4. Fourth Dorsal Web (Chyu-chyo, Chung-chu) Figure 52a.
   Between fourth and fifth dorsal metacarpal phalangeal joints.

XXIII. *Tic Dolereaux* (Trigeminal neuralgia) Second and Third divisions involved.

1. High Lateral Trapezius (Fuchi, Feng-chih) Figure 44b.
   Between trapezius muscle and mastoid process.
2. Fifth Dorsal Metacarpal (kokei, Hon-chi) Figure 53.
   Make a fist and find ulnar end of palmar crease.
3. Superior Tragus (Jimon, Erh-men) Figure 38.
   Immediately above tragus.
4. First Dorsal Metacarpal (Gokoku, Ho-ku) Figures 52 a and b.
   Radial volar aspect of the middle portion of the second metacarpal bone.

XXIV. *Urticaria, exzema, pruritis*

1. Lateral Cubital Crease (Kyokuchi, Chu-chih) Figures 54 and 57.
   Flex elbow and radial end of skin crease.
2. Lateral Upper Tibia (Ashi sanri, Tsu-san-li) Figures 60 a and c.

Three fingerbreadths below tibial tuberosity and one fingerbreadth lateral of tibia.

3. First Dorsal Metacarpal (Gokoku, Ho-ku) Figures 52 a and b.
   Radial volar aspect of the middle portion of the second metacarpal bone.
4. Superior Median Patella (Ketsukai) Figure 65.
   Hold patella with the opposite hand. This point is under thumb.

XXV. *Dysmenorrhea*

1. Para L5-S1 (Kangenyu) Figure 51a.
   Two fingerbreadths lateral of L5 and S1.
2. Low Hypogastrium (Kangen, Kun-yuan) Figure 50.
   At midline on a line from pubis to umbilicus, three-fifths distance from umbilicus to pubis.

XXVI. *Cataracts, tearing*

1. Median Canthus (Seimei, Ching-ming) Figure 40.
   Upper median of canthus inner edge of orbital bone.
   Caution: Might damage lacrimal duct.
2. Lateral Infraorbital (Kyugo, Chiu-hon) Figure 41.
   One-third distance of a line from lateral to median corner of eye on the infraorbital ridge between eyeball and orbit.
3. Inframastoid (Imei, I-ming) Figure 43.
   Just below mastoid.
   Caution: Facial nerve exists from skull close to this location.

XXVII. *Optic nerve atrophy, glaucoma*

1. Lateral Infraorbital (Kyugo, Chiu-hon) Figure 41.
   One-third distance of a line from lateral to median corner of eye on the infraorbital ridge between eye ball and orbit.
2. High Lateral Trapezius (Fuchi, Feng-chih) Figures 44 a and b.
   Between trapezius muscle and mastoid process.
3. Medial Canthus (Seimei, Ching-ming) Figure 40.
   Upper median of canthus inner edge of orbital bone.
4. Inframastoid (Imei, I-ming) Figure 43.
   Just below mastoid.
   Caution: Facial nerve exists from skull close to this location.

XXVIII. *Rhinitis*

1. Glabella (Indo, Yie-tang) Figure 38.
   Between two eyebrows above nasion.
2. First Dorsal Metacarpal (Gokoku, Ho-ku) Figures 52 a and b.

Radial volar aspect of the middle portion of the second metacarpal bone.

XXIX. *Myopia*

1. Mid Infraorbital (Shyokyu, Cheng-chi) Figure 40.
   Just above midpoint of the inferior orbital ridge.
2. Lateral Infraorbital (Kyugo, Chiu-hon) Figure 40.
   One-third distance of a line from lateral to median corner.
3. Medial Canthus (Seimei, Ching-ming) Figure 40.
   Upper median of canthus inner edge of orbital bone.
4. Inframastoid (Imei, Feng-chih)
   Just below mastoid.
   Caution: Facial nerve exists from skull close to this location.
5. High Lateral Trapezius (Fuchi, Feng-chih) Figures 44 a and b.
   Between trapezius muscle and mastoid process.

CHAPTER 3

ACUPUNCTURE ANESTHESIA

DESPITE THE LONG HISTORY OF acupuncture for various ailments, use of acupuncture for anesthesia is quite new even in China. The successful use of acupuncture for prevention of pain during dressing changes in Shanghei Hospital was followed by the successful use of acupuncture for prevention of post tonsilectomy pain.[67] Thus, acupuncture was further advanced as a means of anesthesia. This chapter is based on the information reported by Japanese physicians who visited the Peoples' Republic of China, and our experimental knowledge of acupuncture anesthesia.

In 1970, a total of 400,000 acupuncture anesthesia cases had been reported in the Peoples' Republic of China. This modality has been used for patients aged two days to eighty-one years for major and minor surgical cases and in 250 different types of operations with 90 percent success. Development of acupuncture anesthesia was considered not as an independent aspect of anesthesia but as a tool to improve the current anesthesia. It is important to know, however, that the ratio of acupuncture anesthesia to all anesthesia cases was said to be 10 to 30 percent, although it was 60 percent in the early times of acupuncture anesthesia.

It has been reported that indications for acupuncture anesthesia include the patient's desire, the patient's general condition, and the type of operation. Close relationship between the patient and anesthesiologist developed during a four to five day preoperative period. In general, the success rate is said to be higher in patients over sixty years of age, who have a higher risk with regular anesthesia. This may be due to a decrease in their sensory reactivity. In general, Opistan (25-100 mg) and phenobarbital (100 mg) have been used routinely prior to acupuncture anesthesia.[67]

ADVANTAGES AND DISADVANTAGES OF ACUPUNCTURE ANESTHESIA

Advantages

Consciousness. The physiologic function is unaltered; besides lack of pain sensation, the patient has clear consciousness, hemodynamics, metabolic, respiratory, digestive and neuromotor functions. In addition, needle stimulation to a meridian point is said to harmonize an ill condition positively toward recovery.

During surgery, the patient is able to assist the surgeon by communicating and moving his extremities as directed by the surgeon. For example, a patient could speak during throidectomy and help to prevent accidental damage to the recurrent laryngeal nerve.

Minimum postoperative pain and quick recovery. Postoperative pain is less severe. There is no limitation to motor or digestive functions. The patient is able to have early ambulation and oral feeding. If the patient complains of pain a few hours after surgery, acupuncture anesthesia may be repeated.

Minimum side effects.

Simple, economical and easy to learn. Acupuncture anesthesia requires a minimum of equipment and is reasonably economical. Training for acupuncture anesthesia only requires the knowledge of the location of meridian points and their effects. A practical exercise usually takes not more than one month to learn.

Disadvantages

It has been pointed out that there are cases with incomplete anesthesia with or without nausea and vomiting. No muscle relaxation may be obtained during the procedure.

PATHOPHYSIOLOGY

According to reports from the Peoples' Republic of China, pathophysiology of acupuncture anesthesia is explained as follows:

Needle feeling or *needle shock,* which is a dull radiating aching when proper acupuncture is given, provides specific sensory impulses to the brain. Pain due to surgery and the specific impulse due to the needle oppose each other at a nonspecific projection system in the cerebrum. The impulse due to acupuncture is thought to occupy a main area of the brain and repel pain, due to surgery, to a nonessential area of the brain. This eventually stops the pain sensation and forms an anesthetic state.[67] The mechanism then requires (1) absolutely normal physiologic function of the brain, and (2) an acceptable volume of stimulation continued for a certain period of time.

Conduction of needle feeling impulses is thought to be by two routes. One is through Meridian Points which correspond to the peripheral somatic nervous system; the other is by Meridian Lines which are felt to be autonomic nerve fibers contained in blood vessels, fascia, tendons and other tissue. The *needle feeling impulse* opposes pain caused by surgery not only in the brain but also in nerve tracts and establishes an anesthetic action. In addition to the anesthetic effect, the *needle feeling impulse* is thought to harmonize various *unbalances* in the patient.

In order to create the best effect, it is essential to provide *the maximum needle feeling* and to evoke minimum surgical pain. This requires of the surgeon speed and accuracy in his surgical procedures. It is therefore required to develop close relationships between patient, surgeon, anesthetist and nurses. So it is recommended to call this technique *the operative method with acupuncture anesthesia* rather than simply *acupuncture anesthesia*.[68]

PROCEDURE

Preoperative Preparation

It is essential to obtain excellent communications between patient, medical and paramedical personnel in order to make the patient aggressively cooperative. This includes:

1. adequate explanation of the surgery and anesthesia;
2. preoperative practice of acupuncture anesthesia and analgesia;
3. clear marking of the operative field and the specific meridian points to be used;
4. respiratory exercises, if necessary, in order to prevent mediasitinal flutter;
5. occasional premedication—not necessary in all cases. (Demerol® 50 mg, phenobarbital 100 mg, and atropine 0.5 mg).

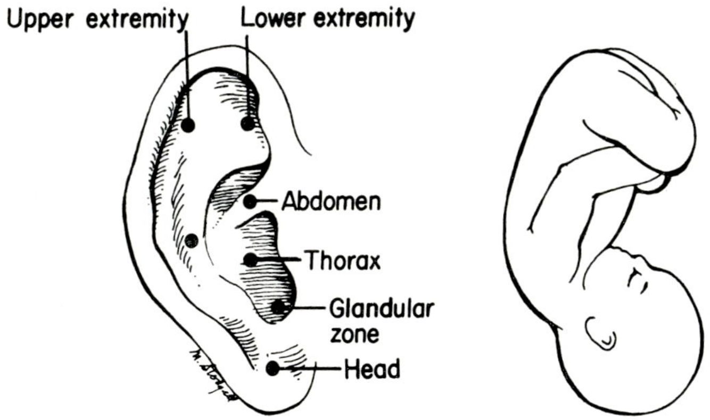

Figure 76: Ear Diagnosis relates to physical abnormality by tenderness on the specific point of the ear. In addition, it has been said that the skin resistance on the particular point of the ear is reduced when the person is ill. The specific points of the ear could be used for acupuncture by using a retention needle 5 mm in depth for 10 minutes. This has been used for static neurolgia and chronic gastritis. However, ear diagnosis is used as an ancillary method for the basic needle therapy. It is believed that acupuncture on the specific point on the ear stabilized autonomic nerve system unbalance.

Selection of the Acupuncture Points

Points are selected by stimulating with finger pressure or acupuncture needles. There are two kinds of points; one is obtained through the meridian line theory and the other new points are obtained from newer experiences and anatomical background (unusual points). There are five methods of technique, the choice of which depends upon where the needles are placed. These are body needles, face needles, ear needles (Fig. 76) nose needles and the hand needles (Table IV). The ear needles and body needles are the only two commonly used.[2]

1. Body Needles
   a. Selection of points based on the meridian line theory.

TABLE IV

Selection for Specific Points in English (Chinese, Japanese)

Operative Field	*Main Points*	*Combination Points*
Head	First dorsal web (hoku, gokoku)	1. High lateral trapezius (feng-chi, fuchi) 2. Infra mastoid (jen-chung, imei)
Eye	First dorsal web (hoku, gokoku)	1. Supraorbital (yang-pe, yokaku) 2. Glabella (yin-tang, taiyo) 3. Temporal (tai-yang, taiyo)
Nose	First dorsal web (hoku, gokoku)	1. Glabella (yin-tang, indu)
Mouth	First dorsal web (hoku, gokoku)	1. Lateral oral angle (ti-ts'ang, chiso) 2. Inferior masseter (chia-che, kyoshaya)
Cheek	First dorsal web (hoku, gokoku)	1. Lateral oral angle (ti-ts'ang, chiso) 2. Inferior masseter (chia-che, kyoshaya) 3. Infratemporal (hsia-kuan, naikan)
Pharynx	First dorsal web (hoku, gokoku)	1. Volar distal forearm (nei-kuan, naikan)
Neck	First dorsal web (hoku, gokoku)	1. Volar distal forearm (nei-kuan, naikan)
Chest	First dorsal web (hoku, gokoku)	1. Volar distal forearm (nei-kuan, naikan)
Lung	First dorsal web (hoku, gokoku)	1. Volar distal forearm (nei-kuan, naikan)
Abdomen	First dorsal web (hoku, gokoku)	1. Volar distal forearm (nei-kuan, naikan)
Stomach	First dorsal web (hoku, gokoku)	1. Volar distal forearm (nei-kuan, naikan) 2. Lateral upper tibia (tsu-san-li, ashi sanri)
Pancreas	First dorsal web (hoku, gokoku)	1. Volar distal forearm (nei-kuan, naikan)
Appendix	First dorsal web (hoku, gokoku)	1. Volar distal forearm (nei-kuan, naikan)
Hernia	First dorsal web (hoku, gokoku)	1. Volar distal forearm (nei-kuan, naikan) 2. Posterior low tibia (san-yin-chiao, saninko) 3. Anterior upper fibula (yang-lin-chuan, yuryosen)
Bladder	Posterior low tibia (san-yin-chiao, saninko)	1. Low hypogastrium (kuan-yuan, kangen)
Uterus	Lateral upper tibia (tsu-san-li, ashi-sanri)	1. Posterior low tibia (san-yin-chiao, saninko)
Ovaries	Posterior low tibia (san-yin-chiao, saninko)	
Upper Arm	First dorsal web (hoku, gokoku) Lateral cubital crease (chu-chih, kyo-ku-chi)	1. Volar distal forearm (nei-kuan, naikan) 2. Dorsal upper forearm (szu-tu, shitoku)
Hand	First dorsal web (hoku, gokoku) Lateral cubital crease (chu-chih, kyo-ku-chi)	1. Fourth dorsal web (chung-chu, chyuchyo)

Select those which provide effective needle feeling in the meridian system controlling the operative area.
For example, lateral upper tibia (ashi sanri, tsu-san-li) for appendectomy, and first dorsal web (gokoku, hoku), lateral cubital crease (kyoku chi, chu-chih) for surgery of thumb and index finger.

b. Selection of the points based on the somatic nerve supply.
Obtain the points over the nerve supply which control the operative area.
For example, superficial cervical plexus for surgery of the thyroid. Supra orbital, supratrochlear N for surgery of the head, and infraorbital N or mandibular N for removal of a tooth.

c. Local selection—needles may be applied at the site of the incision wound with electric current.

d. Symptomatic selection—if the patient pushes during laparotomy, apply a needle at the lateral upper tibia (ashi sanri, tsu-san-li). This may be done according to the traditional acupuncture concept.

2. Ear Needles[68]
   a. Basic Points
   Shinmon for control of cortical stimulation and inhibition of the brain; *lung* for control of the skin area, *sympathetic* for control of the autonomic innervation and relax tonicity of internal organs.
   b. Location of Points
   Anatomically corresponding points of the organ to be operated. For example: keiketsu for thyroidectomy and fukuketsu for appendectomy. If the operative field is at one side of the body, then use the points at the same side of the ear.
   c. Symptomatic Points (according to traditional acupuncture theory)
   Muscle tones for spleen (spleen control muscle), skin for lung (lung control skin), bone for kidney (kidney control bone).
3. *Method of Stimulation*
   a. Needle—stainless steel No. 32 (0.26 mm x 13 mm to 26 mm) for ear needle; No. 28 to 30, (0.32 mm to 0.38 mm x 39mm to 150 mm) for body needle. Specific caution against hepatitis is needed. Needles should be boiled at 100° C for thirty minutes and placed in a 75 percent alcohol solution.
   b. *Techniques*—mental and physical stability of the patient are required in order to obtain the *needle feeling* from the patient. When the patient notices the *needle feeling* then the needle should be advanced a little. Angle the needle at 90° against the skin. Ear needles should be placed directly or obliquely so it does not

penetrate the opposite skin. Occasionally place one needle to two points by penetrating one point to the other.

1. Hand motion—degree of stimulation may be changed by finger manipulation, twirling and sparrow pecking motions. Again it is necessary that the manipulation must be light, accurate, calm, and rapid.
2. Specific devices to move a needle—a machine that moves the needle up and down or twirls the needle.
3. Electric Acupuncture—square shaped wave is used (10 to 60 volts, 180 to 200 cycles per minute). Frequency and amperage should be changed during procedure. D.C. current should not be used since this current causes skin burns and electrical disassociation.
4. Water needle—5 percent dextrose in water, 0.9 percent normal saline, procaine or vitamin B solution may be used, 0.1 to 0.211 for ear needles and 3 to 10 cc. for body needles. This requires twenty minutes for onset of effect and to maintain the effect for one hour.
5. Finger pressure—compress the acupuncture points for one to three minutes then operative field should also be compressed.
6. Combination of the above.

c. *Chinese Model 71-1 Acupuncture Anesthesia Apparatus*[69] (Fig. 77). This portable type apparatus may be used for acupuncture

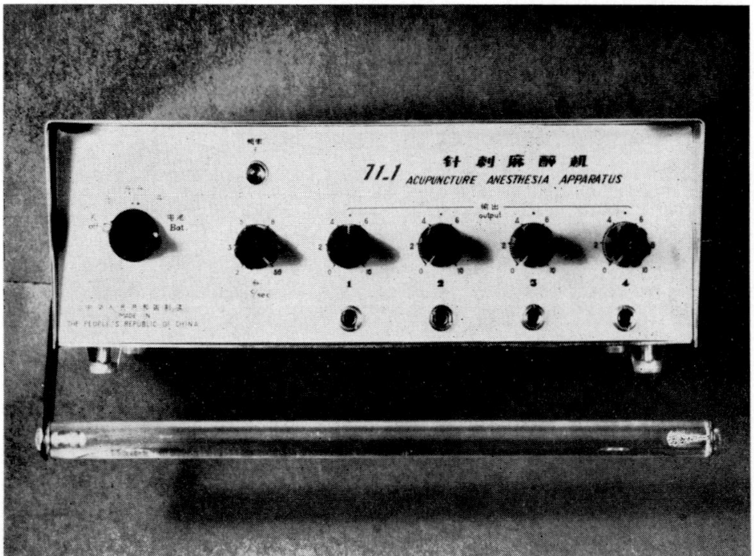

Figure 77: Acupuncture anesthesia apparatus made in the People's Republic of China.

anesthesia and electrotherapeutic stimulation according to their description. The nervous or muscular system is excited for therapeutic purposes and inhibited for anesthetic purposes by means of stimulation.

1) *Range of Application*

   The application can improve peripheral circulation and adjust the tonicity of the nervous and muscular system. In addition, the apparatus is reported to be useful in treatment of contusion, sprain, arthritis, sore legs and tenosynobitis.

2) *Direction for Operation*

   a) Turn changing switch to required wave.
   b) Illumination on the frequency pilot light indicates the apparatus is functioning (sending output pulse current).
   c) This apparatus is capable of providing three wave forms.

      (1) "Switch to 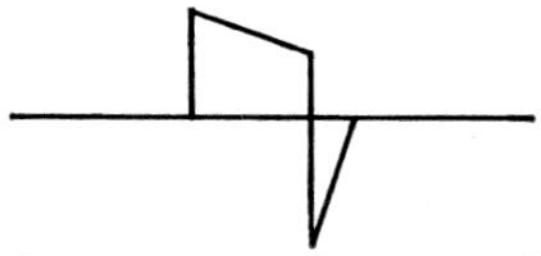 position"

      1, 2, 3, and 4 output sockets produces the same wave

      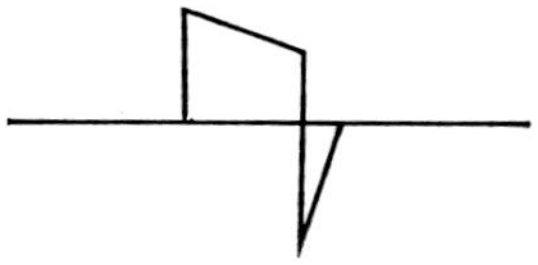

      (2) "Switch to 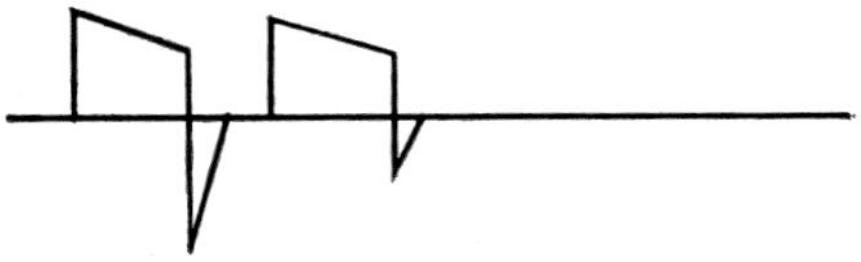 position"

      1, and 2 output socket produces

      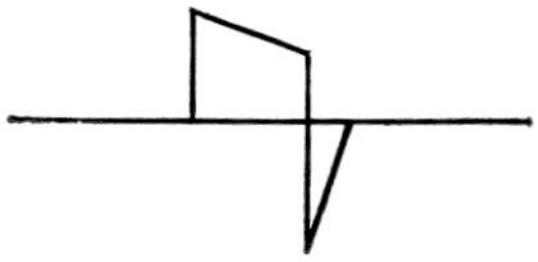 (strong).

      3, and 4 output socket produces

      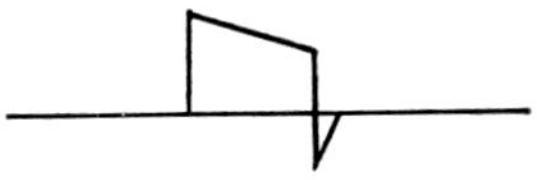 (weak).

      (3) "Switch to 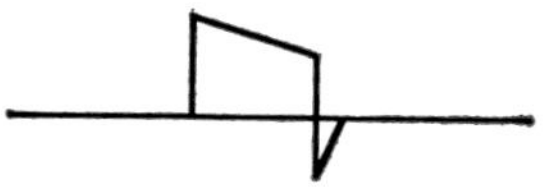 position"

      1, 2, 3, and 4 output socket produces

      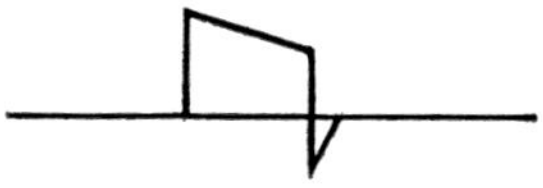

d) Connect the output electrode wave plug to output sockets (1 to 4).
e) Each electrode has two clips which hold acupuncture needles.
f) Thus, total of 4 sets output sockets can afford 8 acupuncture points.
g) Current strength should be adjusted by turning the current regulator.

3) *Power Supply*
D.C. 9 volts, 6 batteries (1.5 volts each).

4) *Notes*
a) When the apparatus is not in use turn the knob to *off*.
b) Brightness of the pilot lamp assists to check the power consumption by turning the changing switch to battery.
c) Efficacy of this apparatus is closely related to the location of needles and experience of physician.

It has been reported that when specific acupuncture points are stimulated with finger motion, EEG revealed sinusoidal wave with less than 8 Hz. When pain is introduced during surgery the EEG reverses to normal alpha rhythm.

In spite of various reports, the patient who underwent thoracotomy had been prepared with pulmonary physical therapy and even with artifical pneumothorax. These preparations are not well known to us. In addition, it is my upmost concern to learn what is the value of blood gasses and degree of pulmonary shunt during the thoracotomy under acupuncture anesthesia.

CHAPTER 4

ACUPUNCTURE RESEARCH

BASIC STUDY

A *Histologic changes following acupuncture* (studied and prepared by Mr. R. Weiss):

Acupuncture with a No. 3 needle (diameter 0.24 mm) into animal muscles and nerves injured an average of seven to twelve fibers and eight to fifteen nerve fibers respectively (Fig. 78-81).

b. *Bacteriologic study of acupuncture needles:*

Seven acupuncture needles were contaminated with various bacteria (pseudomonas, krebsiella and E. coli) and wiped once with a dry sponge (Fig. 17). The needles were then cultured and it was found that no organism could be isolated (Fig. 18).

c. *Microcirculatory responses following acupuncture:*

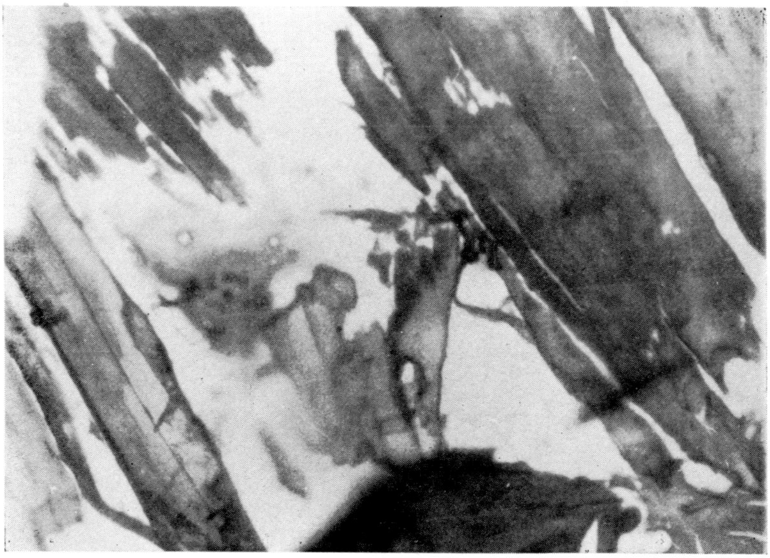

Figure 78: Figure destruction immediately after sparrow pecking motion (10 times with 25 gauge hypodermic needle).

The Research, reported in this chapter was carried out by the author.

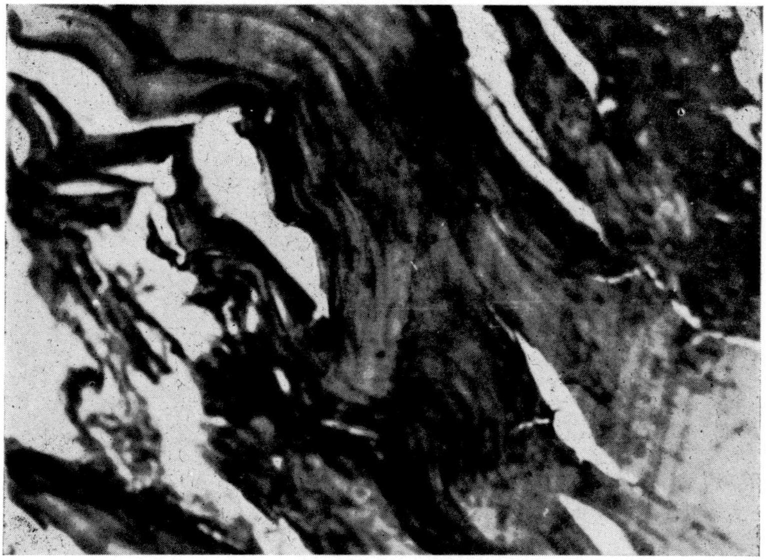

Figure 79: Same above, 10 days later.

Microcirculatory responses of various organs were evaluated and it was found that the acupuncture given at the second interdigital web space of the forepaw produced relative vasoconstriction followed by vasodilation in the splanchinic vessels.

d. *Acupuncture and intestinal motility* (prepared by Dr. V. Ambruso):

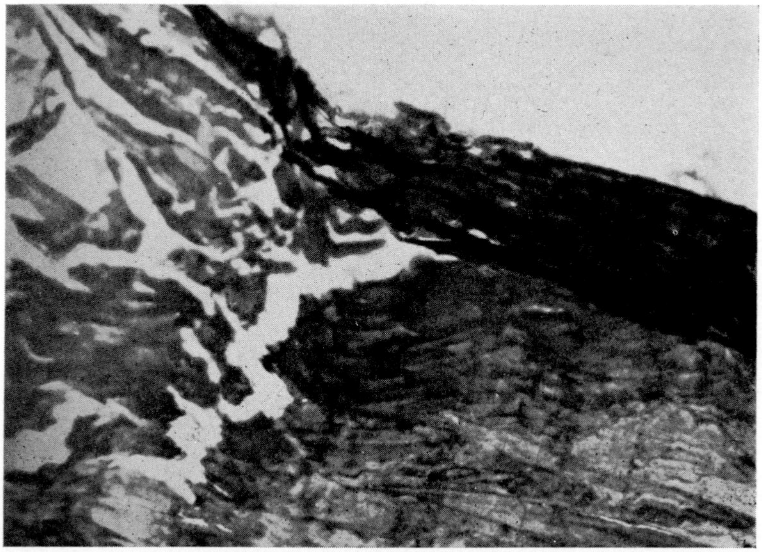

Figure 80: Muscle destruction immediately after sparrow pecking motion (100 times with a No. 3 acupuncture needle).

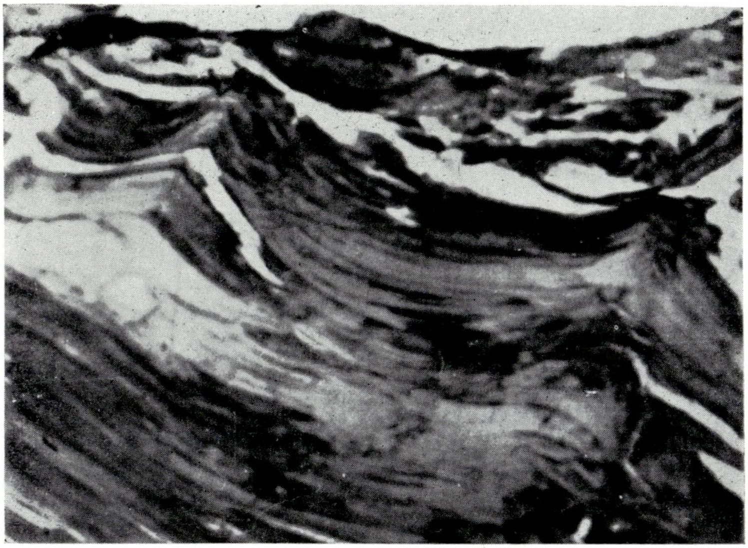

Figure 81: Same above, 10 days later.

The objective of this study was to evaluate the efficacy of electric stimulation in the management of gastrointestinal atony.

Sixty rabbits and ten patients were studied. In the rabbits, two balloon catheters were placed in the small and large bowel and calibrated to record pressure (Fig. 82). Each animal served as its own control. EEG, EKG, arterial blood pressure, and respiration rate were simultaneously recorded. The positive terminal was applied to the vertex, thumb, index of the first toe or second tow web. Right groin was used as the negative terminal. The motility curve was allowed to return to the baseline before continuing to the next experiment. Animals were equally divided into three groups according to stimulus: Group 1, Sine Wave; Group 2, Delta Wave; Group 3, Square Wave. Patients with laparotomies were divided equally into two groups. Upper lateral tibial point (Sanri) was selected for insertion of needles. While Group 1 received electric current, (Sine Wave 200 microamperes 10 K Hertz with the negative terminal at the right thumb web) Group 2 received no stimulation. Amplitude and frequency of intestinal motility curve in control were 3 to 5 cm H_2O and 2 to 5 contractions per forty second intervals. The best results were obtained when sine wave was applied to the index web which recorded 20 to 30 cm H_2O and nine to eighteen contractions per forty seconds (Fig. 83 and 84). The delta and square wave resulted in no difference from the control recordings. In all rabbits, peristalsis became visible in fifteen minutes after acupuncture and defecation developed within thirty minutes after acupuncture. No changes in the other measured parameter where noted except for increased alpha and occasional delta waves in EEG. In acupuncture patients, immediate relief of abdominal distension

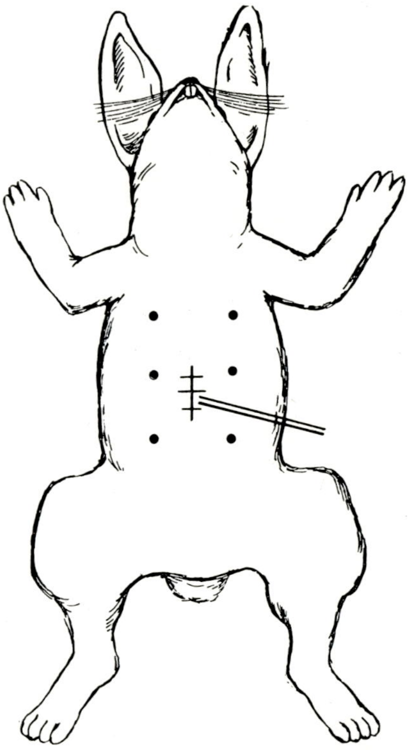

Figure 82: Balloon catheter was placed in the small bowel and calibrated to record pressure.

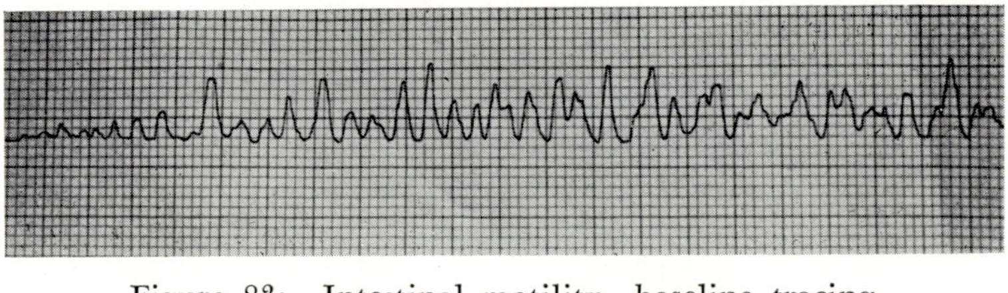

Figure 83: Intestinal motility—baseline tracing.

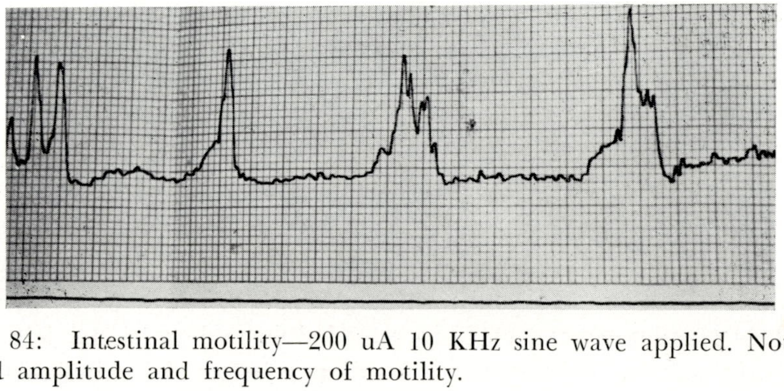

Figure 84: Intestinal motility—200 uA 10 KHz sine wave applied. Note: Increased amplitude and frequency of motility.

and pain were noted and defecation followed within twenty-four hours while no defecation was noted in an average of seventy-two hours when acupuncture was not given.

e. *Responses of experimentally induced inflammatory joint to acupuncture.* (Conducted and prepared by Dr. E. Marmar)

This study was designed to elucidate the effects of acupuncture as they relate to acute infammation.

Acupuncture stimulation was given to groups of five Wister male albino rats, with either normal or carrageenin inflamed paws, according to one of the following schedules: one ten minute treatment (Schedule A); five 30 second treatments given hourly (Schedule B); or three 30 second treatments given at the outset, one and four hours later (Schedule C). Acupuncture needles were inserted at the specific acupuncture points on the paw or knee which were located by a galvanometer as spots of lowered electrical skin resistance. Plethysmographic measurement of the paw volumes was done hourly for five hours and twenty-four hours after the initial baseline reading. A mean paw volume increase of 4 to 14 percent developed in fifteen rats stimulated at the paw acupuncture point. This persisted twenty-four hours in the ten rats receiving stimulation according to Schedules B and C. Stimulation at the paw point of ten rats, according to Schedules B and C, given post inflammation caused an average 20 percent ($p<0.05$) suppression of the carrageenin response twenty-four hours after injection of the edemogen. Stimulation at the knee point created minimal inflammation in fifteen normal rats. Fifteen rats with carrageenin edema given Schedule A pre and post inflammation and Schedule C post inflammation at the knee point, developed a 15 to 25 percent ($p<0.05$) increase over control edema at the twenty-four measurement.

Acupuncture stimulation created a local inflammation which persists for twenty-four hours when multiple treatments were given. Multiple acupuncture stimulation given locally had an anti-inflammatory effect, while distant acupuncture stimulation had an enhancing effect on the course of carrageenin edema.

EXPERIMENTAL ACUPUNCTURE ANESTHESIA (Selection of Optimal Electric Current)

Despite nearly three thousand years experience with acupuncture for pain relief and treatment of various pathologic conditions, the concept of acupuncture anesthesia is relatively new even to the Chinese. Reports from China have been very fragmentary and technical details and controlled studies are sparse despite Chinese information that nearly one half million procedures have been performed using acupuncture anesthesia as the sole analgesic modality.

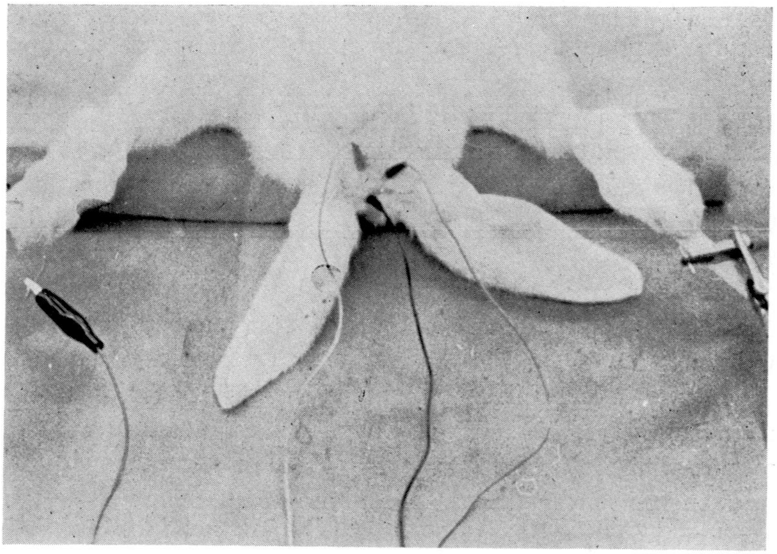

Figure 85: Rabbit was restrained in a supine position and three scalp electrodes for electroencephalogram were attached. In this figure, an acupuncture needle was placed in second interdigital space bilatreally.

The objective of this study was to evaluate the type of stimulation to be used in order to obtain optimal results with acupuncture anesthesia.

Materials and Methods

For our studies of acupuncture anesthesia a specific laboratory was kept dark and quiet. The same technicians were assigned to the entire study and had free access to the opinions of consultant neurologists and bioengineers.

Forty-four rabbits were utilized as study subjects. They were shaved, restrained in a supine position and prepared by attaching three subcortical electrodes (frontal, parietal and occipital) for electroencephalogram (EEG) recording (Fig. 85). A reference electrode was placed on the anterior center of the rabbit's thigh. A Grass polygraph machine was then prepared to chart the EEG at prescribed settings. (Paper speed 24 mm/sec, sensitivity 75 uV/cm, 60 ohm filter was used, range of frequency was ½ amp low—1, and ½ amp high—15) (Fig. 86). EEG readings were standardized by response of the animals to pain produced by externally applied stimuli. An acupuncture needle was placed in second interdigital web spaces of an upper or lower paw to a depth of 3 centimeters between bones.

A signal generator was then set to produce a desired frequency and wave form (Fig. 87). The circuit was then completed by attaching the anodal lead of the generator to the acupuncture needle and the cathodal

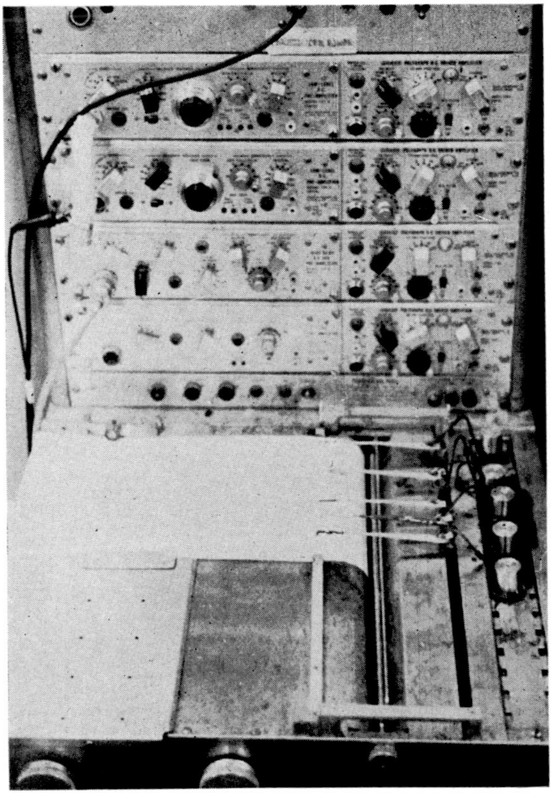

Figure 86: Grass Polygraph machine was prepared to chart the EEG at prescribed setting.

lead to a preset resistor (Fig. 88) which was connected to the rabbit at its thigh by means of a 20 gauge stainless steel needle. An oscilloscope was then used to measure voltage across both the resistor and the entire circuit. Thus, one was able to determine amperage by using Ohm's law.

Any desired amperage could be obtained by then resetting the signal generator and measuring the current with the oscilloscope, providing the requisite voltage was less than thirty which was the maximum capability of our generator. After each hour of stimulation, the circuit was disconnected and the rabbit's EEG was read after various stimuli to the rabbit. Upon completion of this charting, the rabbit was again returned to the circuit at the preset amperage. Animals were evaluated for anesthesia by Kocher clamping of the entire body surface. An area of anesthesia was determined by lack of animal pain response (motion, cried) and EEG findings revealing no peak wave phenomenon.

A body map of anesthetized arrears was made every thirty minutes for a six hour period.

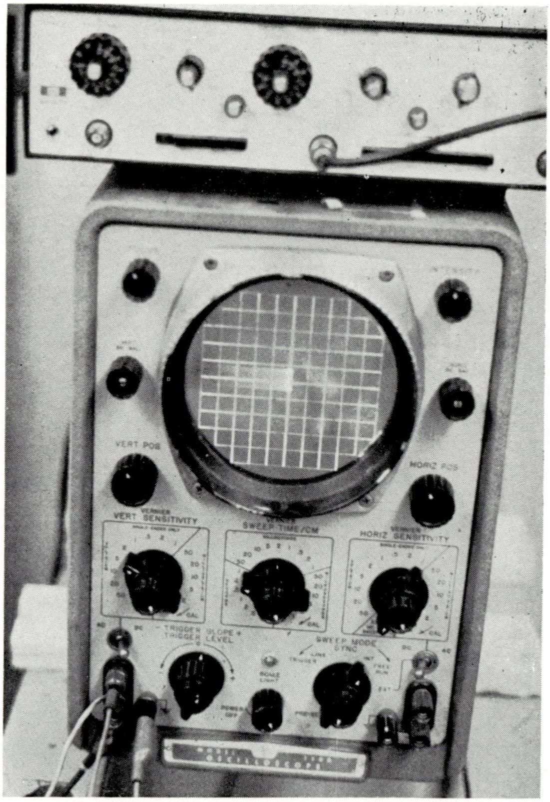

Figure 87: A signal generator was set to produce a desired frequency and wave form. An oscilloscope was used to measure voltage across both the resistor and the entire circuit.

Complete blood count and biochemical profile were studied before and at termination of acupuncture anesthesia. Careful evaluation of EEG response, EEG amplitude, EEG frequency, motion of animal, cries, pulse rate, respiration and eye signs was performed every thirty minutes before, during and after discontinuation of electric current until complete recovery sensation to the anesthetized region.

The animals were divided into six groups:

Group 1 (4 rabbits): Control:
Animals were kept in a supine position for six hours. An acupuncture needle was placed but no electric current was given.

Group 2 (8 rabbits): Current (Different Amperage):
In this group of rabbits, square wave (pulse length, 1 milli-second, 100 cycles per second) was used. Acu-

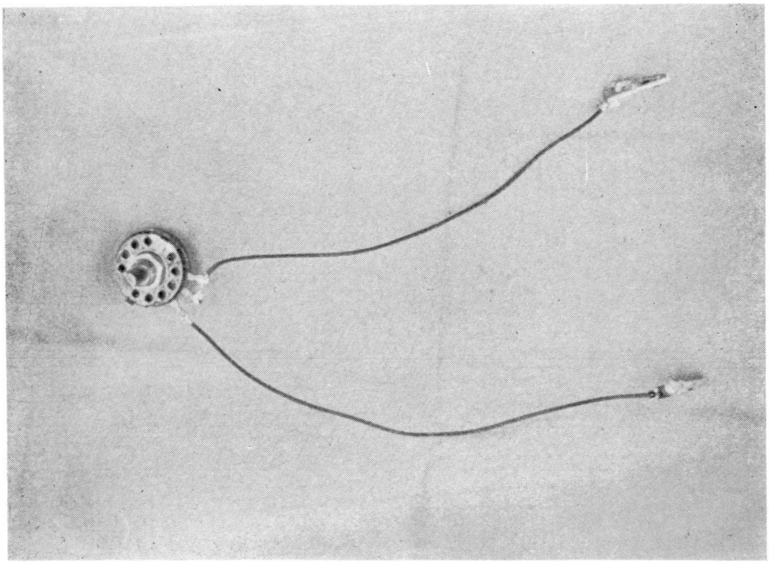

Figure 88: Resistor

puncture needle was placed at the second interdigital space of right upper paw. On six rabbits of subgroup 1, 200 microamperes of electric current was applied, while 500 microamperes was applied in two rabbits of subgroup 2.

Group 3 (10 rabbits): Location of Acupuncture Needles:
In this group, the same electric current (pulse length 1 millisecond, 100 cycles per second) as was applied in subgroup 1 of Group 2 was used. However, an acupuncture needle was placed at the third interdigital space of the right upper paw in two rabbits of subgroup 1; fourth interdigital space of right upper paw in 2 rabbits of subgroup 2 and second interdigital space of left lower paw in two rabbits in subgroup 3, third interdigital space of left lower paw in two rabbits of subgroup 4, and fourth interdigital space of left lower paw in two rabbits of subgroup 5.

Group 4 (8 rabbits): Wave Forms:
In this group of rabbits an acupuncture needle was placed in the second interdigital space of the upper right paw as in subgroup 1 of Group 2. In two rabbits of subgroup 2 triangle shaped wave was applied.

In each subgroup, 200 microamperes of current with 100 cycles per second was used. In two rabbits of subgroup 1, a delta shaped wave was used.

Group 5 (8 rabbits): Cycles:
In this group, all rabbits received 200 microamperes sine wave current to an acupuncture needle in the second interdigital space of the upper right paw. In subgroup 1 of two rabbits 1 cycle per second was used. In subgroup 2 of two rabbits, 1000 cycles per second was used. In subgroup 3 of two rabbits 10,000 cycles per second and in subgroup 4 of two rabbits 100,000 cyces per second was used.

Group 6 (6 rabbits): Manual Stimulation:
In this group a needle was placed at the second interdigital space of the right upper paw and a needle was manually twirled continuously.

Results

In animals in group 1, it was learned that the animals would move vigorously and cry when the Kocher clamp was applied to the skin without acupuncture anesthesia, in addition, pulse rate increased. Figure 89 shows the EEG on the unanesthetized animal with characteristic beta waves of 18

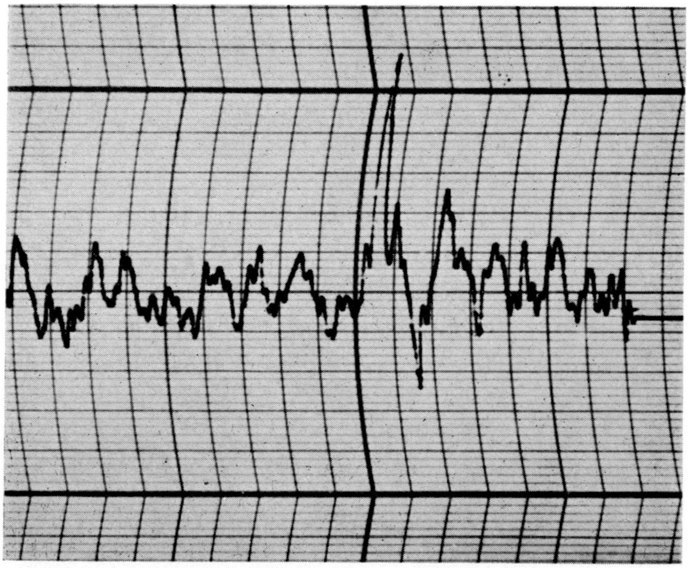

Figure 89: EEG of animal kept six hours in a supine position revealed peak wave immediately after stimulation on abdominal wall.

to 25 per second frequency. When the Kocher clamp was applied to the skin, the EEG revealed a sharp wave which was a typical pain response in the unanesthetized animal. In addition, pulse rate was increased. In our study, the calculated skin resistance of rabbits was approximately 3,000 OHM's measured between right thigh and the paw of right upper leg.

In animals in Group 2, the initial area of anesthesia was the mid-anterior chest only. This area of anesthesia further increased to the abdominal area and laterally in a matter of time. It was apparent that as the period of application became longer, the area of anesthesia became wider (Fig. 90). When electric current was increased the area of anesthesia was similar to that seen with lesser electric current but the effect was obtained in less time.

When the skin was anesthetized with acupuncture anesthesia, the animal did not move or cry when the Kocher clamp was applied. In addition, the EEG did not reveal any sharp peak wave (Fig. 91) and no change in pulse rate or eye signs were noted.

In Group 3, the best results were obtained when a needle was placed at the second interdigital space of the upper paw.

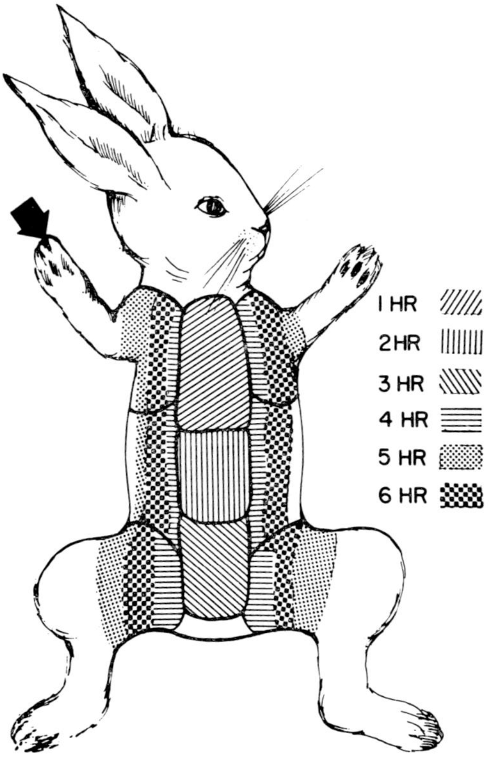

Figure 90: Period of acupuncture anesthesia became longer; the area of anesthesia became wider.

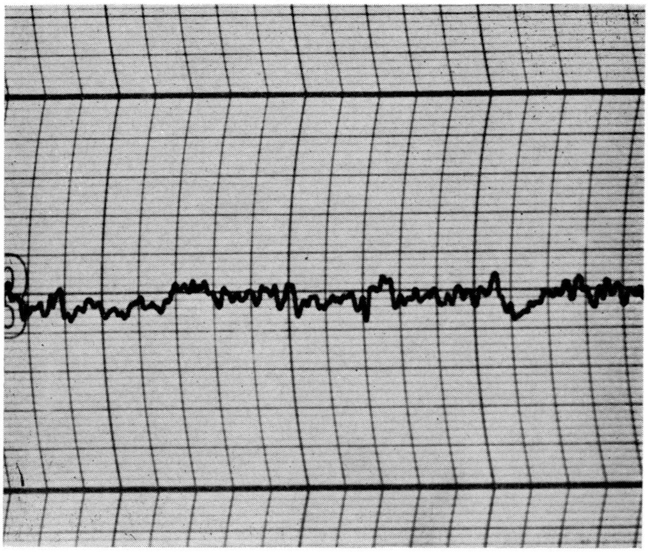

Figure 91: EEG of animal after proper acupuncture anesthesia revealed no response after stimulation of anesthetized area. Note also wave with lesser frequency and lower amplitude compared to the EEG wave in Figure 79.

In Group 4, the best results were obtained with sine wave current (Fig. 92) while delta wave current gave the poorest results (Fig. 93).

In Group 5 when 10,000 cycles per second of sine wave current was used, an area of anesthesia similar to that seen with 100 cycles of sine wave current was obtained in only thirty minutes rather than five hours. As far as frequency is concerned, the higher the frequency the better the results up to 10,000 cycles per second. 100,000 cyces per second did not produce the better effect compared to that with 10,000 cycles/second.

In Group 6, when an acupuncture needle was applied in second interdigital space and manually stimulated, the area of anesthesia was significantly less than that with electric acupuncture.

It was possible to perform surgical procedures on rabbits under the effect of acupuncture anesthesia without any premedication (Fig. 94). Rabbits were able to stand up immediately after discontinuation of electric anesthesia (Fig. 95). No changes in hemodynamics (blood pressure, pulse rate) and eye signs (size of pupils, reaction to light, tearing and eye movement) were noted. In all animals, the area of anesthesia rapidly reduced in an opposite pattern to its induction. When electric acupuncture was discontinued, post-treatment study including gross observation and CBC indicated no evidence of pathology up to two months.

Comment

Despite limited scientific information concerning electric acupuncture

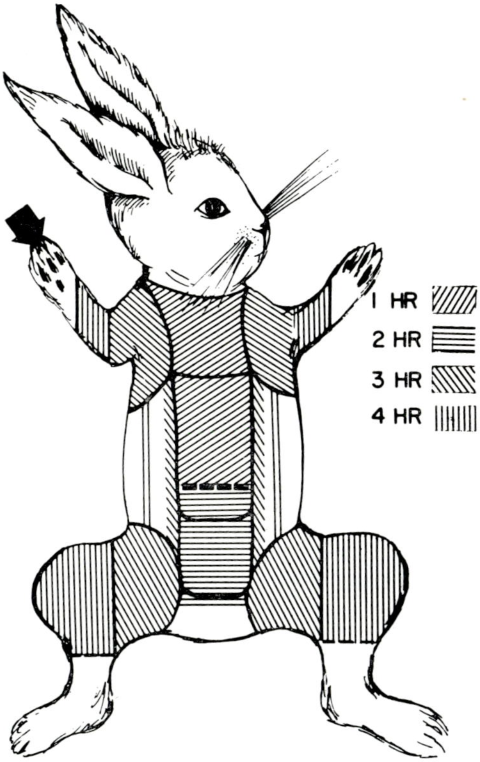

Figure 92: The best results were obtained with sine wave current. When 10,000 cycle per second of sine wave was used, the area of anesthesia similar to this figure (with 100 cycle per second of sine wave) was obtained within 50 minutes instead of five hours.

anesthesia from the Peoples' Republic of China, data from electroanesthesia as used in other medical centers has supplied valuable information. Electric current applied on the nervous system induced a degree of analgesia which was sufficient for delivery. It was reported that the low intensity current applied in this study was not noxious for the child even when it was applied to the mother for as long as three hours.[70]

The electrical cardioversion was used for attacks of patoxysma tachycardia and auricular fibrillation under electroanesthesia. It was reported that at the end of electroanesthesia the patient awoke immediately and absence of pain despite the strong electrical charge used for the cardioversion indicated the adequate depth of anesthesia.[71]

A portable battery powered device which produced the anesthesia was developed and successfully used experimentally. This device produced a sine wave oscillation of 700 Hz and had an output of a minimum of 12 volts and 12 milliamperes.[72]

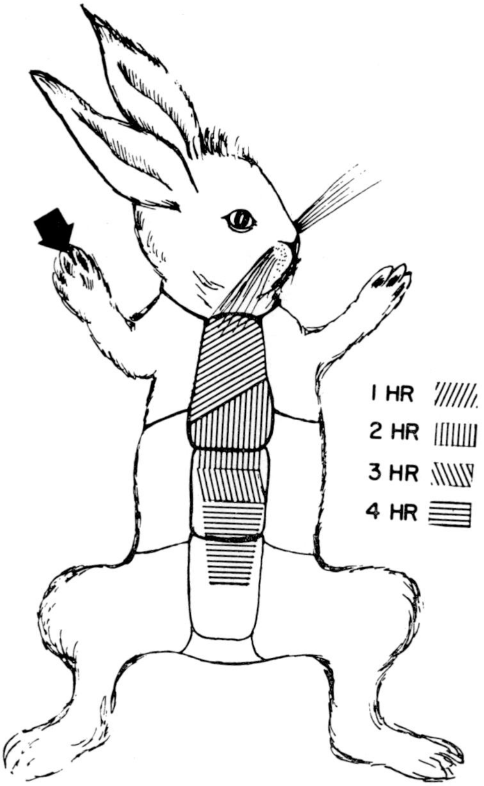

Figure 93: There was a decrease in the area of anesthesia when delta wave current was used.

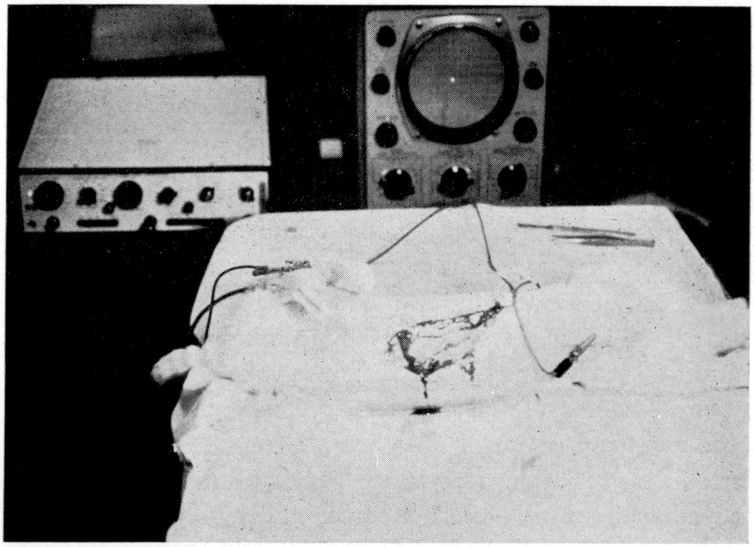

Figure 94: It was possible to perform surgery on rabbits under the effect of acupuncture anesthesia without premedication.

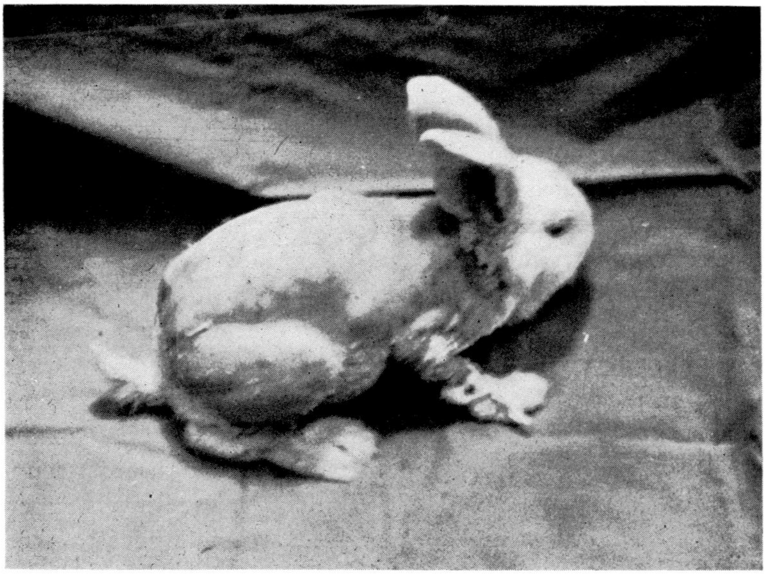

Figure 95: Rabbits were able to stand-up immediately after surgery.

The effect of electroanesthesia upon circulatory serotonin was evaluated. The preliminary findings suggested that changes in serotonin did not play an integral part in the production of electroanesthesia.[73]

Electroanesthesia was used satisfactorily for various surgical procedures in macaca specious monkey. Electroanesthesia was produced by a 70 to 100 Hz rectangular current of 7 milliamperes average 2.5 milli second duration biased 7.0 milliamperes above zero.

The electroanesthesia was reported to be sufficient to produce muscle relaxation and no coughing. Retching and laryngeal spasm were noted. In addition, this study failed to demonstrate marked fluid shift during the application of electroanesthesia.[5]

Another report from Japan indicated that electric acupuncture anesthesia was used in eighty patients. Electric pulses of 60 volts in amplitude with pulse length of 0.1 milliseconds at a rate of one per second were used and continued for four days. It took one hundred minutes to totally anesthetize the patient, excluding the face.[75]

Our studies indicated that routine laboratory animals do not show significant interspecies differences in skin resistance except at small paw and back regions. The study of EEG during acupuncture anesthesia was of great value in the evaluation of acupuncture anesthesia. Peak wave following stimulation is thought to be related to the animal's motion with pain. In this regard, evoked potential study with more sensitive EEG recording now is being started.

However, it is important to know that in our experiment, manual stimulation to the acupuncture needles placed at the specific points, did produce anesthesia without an aid of electric current. Another important factor in acupuncture anesthesia is its distribution. The painless area produced by acupuncture anesthesia is entirely unique and competely different from that produced by regional or spinal block anesthesia. It was learned that the painless area produced was related to many factors, including selection of acupuncture points, type of electric wave and cycle employed. It rather quickly spread from the midline laterally and then to the entire body. More detailed evaluation of the specific point for better anesthesia will be reported in a later chapter. Anesthetic effect was thought to be due to a stimulation not supplied by electric current since stimulation with manual movement of the needles also produced some anesthesia. It is thought that the most effective location for insertion of an acupuncture needle corresponds to an area where a somatic nerve travels superficially.

More detailed study of the specific points in reference to the area of anesthesia will be published separately.

Application of needles at too many acupuncture points on the body surface was found to reduce the effect of anesthesia. In addition, no muscle relaxation was obtained in rabbits in any group by this mode of anesthesia. Continuous DC current appeared not to be effective and high cycle intermittent DC current is now our modality of choice. In this study electric stimulation was used.

It was possible for us to perform surgical procedures on rabbits under the effect of acupuncture anesthesia without any premedication. Thus acupuncture anesthesia may prove valuable in our modern surgery as a type of anesthesia.

Summary

Acupuncture anesthesia was produced in rabbits. The best results were obtained with 200 microamperes, sine wave and 10,000 cycle per second applied to a needle inserted in the second interdigital space of the upper paw when cathodal lead was connected to the rabbit at its thigh.

ACUPUNCTURE ANESTHESIA IN ANIMALS
(Selection of Optimal Specific Locations of Needle Points)

Because of recent public interest in acupuncture for the treatment of chronic pain and also because of its apparent widespread use for anesthesia in the Republic of China, we have been encouraged to study it in a controlled and objective manner in our surgical research laboratories. The objective of this study was to evaluate the efficacy of acupuncture anesthesia in relation to the needle points.

Materials And Methods

Thirty-four medium sized domesticated rabbits were utilized. They were comfortably restrained in a supine position and both manual and electrical acupuncture methods were employed. A No. 3 stainless steel acupuncture needle was inserted subcutaneously to a depth of 3 cm. Electrical stimulation was given as a sine wave at 10 KHz and with 200 microamperes current. Electrocardiogram (ECG), blood pressure (BP) and electroencephalogram (EEG) were also continuously monitored. Eye signs were also evaluated.

Each animal was tested for cutaneous anesthesia by pinprick and clamping of the skin with a Kocher clamp. In the areas of anesthesia, there was no response to the painful stimuli. In these areas where there was no anesthesia, the animal cried, moved and a movement artifact was noted on the EEG. The EEG tracings which were performed with percutaneous electrodes revealed a considerable amount of ECG and EMG artifact. However, when the animal felt pain there was a definite and consistently reproducible movement artifact. In future experiments it is planned to place cortical electrodes in the animals and to study other parameters such as sensory evoked potentials.[76]

Each animal served as its own control in that his response to pinprick and Kocher clamping was noted prior to the application of either manual or electrical acupuncture stimuli.

A total of forty-one rabbits were used. Eight animals in Group 1 were stimulated manually while the remaining thirty-three rabbits in Group 2 were stimulated with electric current. Eight rabbits in Group 1 were further subdivided equally into four subgroups according to the location of the stimulating points. Stimulation was given simultaneously at two points on each animal for a period of forty-five minutes to one hour.

Subgroup 1: Bilateral vertex
Subgroup 2: Second web of fore paw and vertex
Subgroup 3: Third web of fore paw and vertex
Subgroup 4: First web of hind paw and vertex

Thirty-three rabbits in Group 2 were further subdivided equally into eleven subgroups according to the location of the stimulating points.

Subgroup 1: Base of ears
Subgroup 2: Second web of fore paw to right thigh
Subgroup 3: Third web of fore paw to vertex
Subgroup 4: Last web of fore paw to vertex
Subgroup 5: Third web of hind paw to vertex
Subgroup 6: Last web of hind paw to vertex
Subgroup 7: Second web of hind paw to vertex

Subgroup 8: Second web of right fore paw to second web of forepaw
Subgroup 9: Second web of fore paw to vertex
Subgroup 10: Vertex to second web of fore paw
Subgroup 11: Vertex to first web of hind paw

Results

Group 1: Manual Stimulation

Subgroup 1: Bilateral Vertex—an area of cutaneous anesthesia over the thorax between the nipple lines (Fig. 96)

Subgroup 2: Simultaneous stimulation of the second web of right forepaw and vertex

Subgroup 3: Simultaneous stimulation of the third web of the right forepaw and vertex. In subgroup 2 and 3 an area of cutaneous anesthesia was obtained over thorax, abdomen, and pubis between the nipple lines (Fig. 97)

Subgroup 4: Simultaneous stimulation of the second web of the right hind paw and vertex. An area of cutaneous anesthesia was obtained over the thorax and abdomen, which extended laterally to the midaxillary lines (Fig. 98).

The major problem with manual stimulation was the lengthy time in-

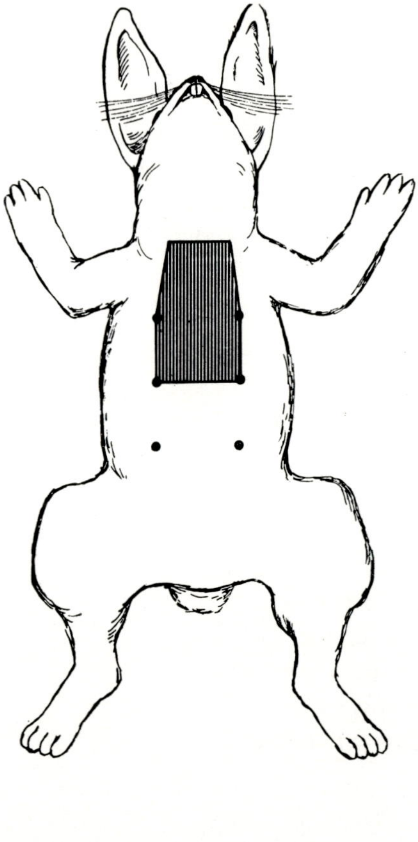

Figure 96: Area of local anesthesia following manual stimulation *bilateral vertex*.

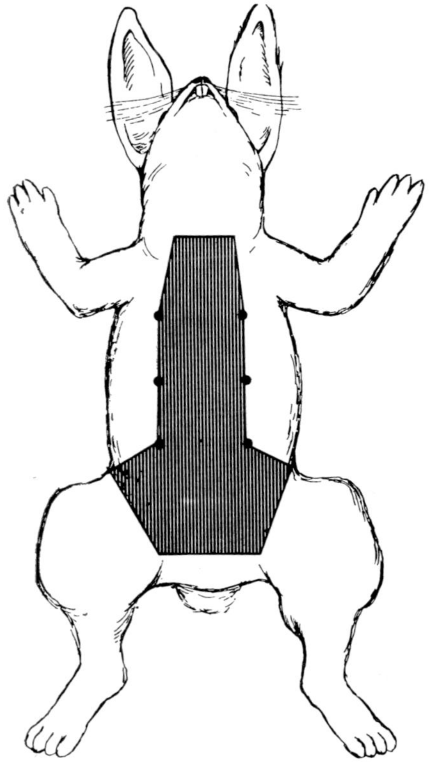

Figure 97: Area of local anesthesia following manual stimulation; "second web of right forepaw and vertex" or "third web of the right forepaw to vertex."

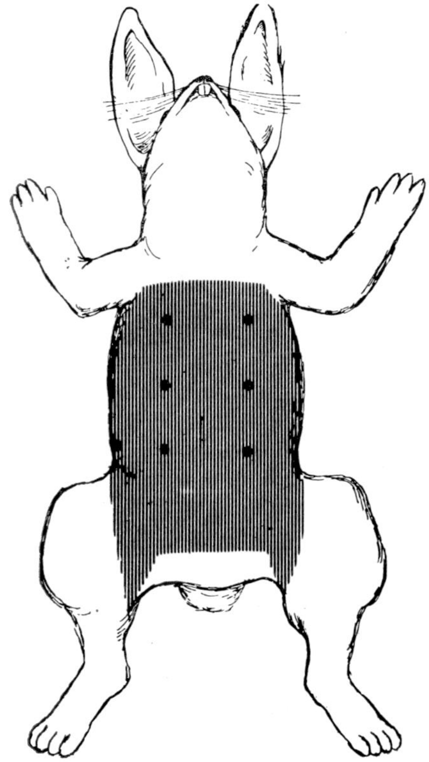

Figure 98: Area of local anesthesia following manual stimulation; "the second web of the right paw and vertex."

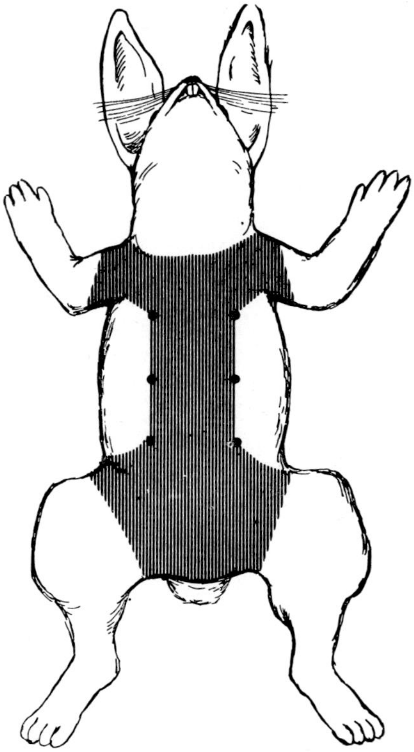

Figure 99: Area of local anesthesia following electric stimulation; "the base of ears."

volved in obtaining cutaneous anesthesia and the loss of anesthesia within a few minutes of cessation of stimulation. However, we were encouraged by the fact that we could induce analgesia by manual manipulation and we undertook the study of electrical stimulation to see if we could not discover a more workable and practical model.

Group 2: Electrical Stimulation (thirty-three animals were utilized)

Subgroup 1: Bilateral parietal electrodes were placed next to each ear along the interaural line. An area of cutaneous analgesia was obtained over thorax, abdomen, and pubis with minimal extension to the axilla and groin bilaterally above and below the nipple line (Fig. 99).

Subgroup 2: Stimulation from second web right fore paw to right thigh. An area of cutaneous analgesia over the thorax and upper abdomen between the nipple lines (Fig. 100).

Subgroup 3: Stimulation from third web of right forepaw to vertex. An area of cutaneous analgesia over thorax and upper abdomen between the nipple lines (Fig. 101).

Subgroup 4: Stimulation from last web of right forepaw to vertex.

Subgroup 5: Stimulation from third web of right hind paw to vertex.

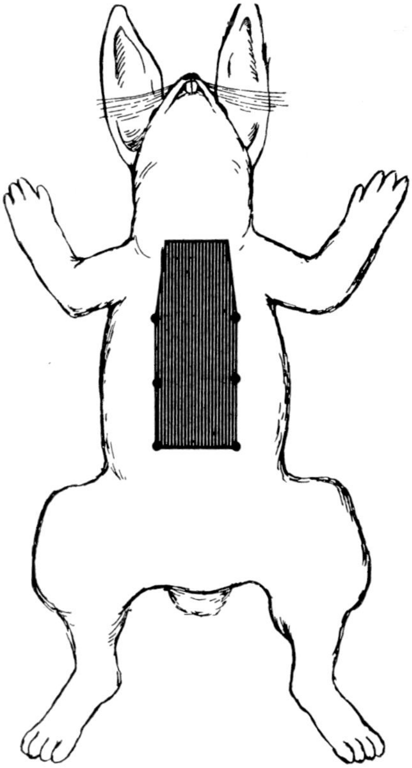

Figure 100: Area of local anesthesia following electric stimulation; "second web of right forepaw to right thigh.

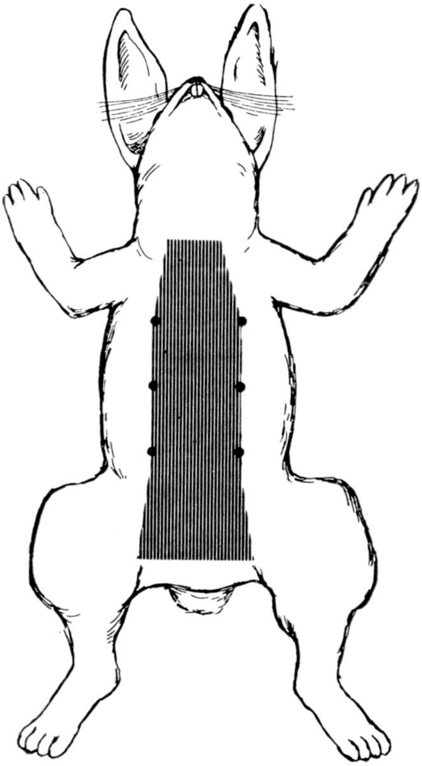

Figure 101: Area of local anesthesia following electric stimulation; "third web of right forepaw to vertex."

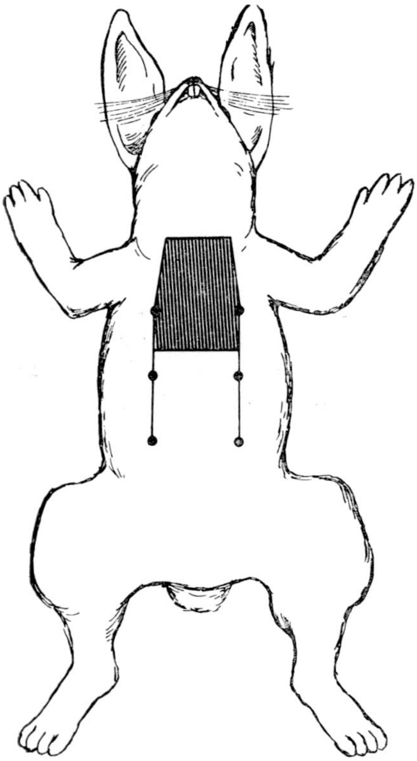

Figure 102: Area of local anesthesia following electric stimulation; "last web of right forepaw to vertex" or "third web of right hind paw to vertex" or "last web of right hind paw to vertex."

Subgroup 6: Stimulation from last web of right hind paw to vertex. An area of cutaneous analgesia over the upper thorax between the nipple lines in subgroup 4, 5, and 6 (Fig. 102).

Subgroup 7: Stimulation from second web of right hind paw to vertex. An area of cutaneous anesthesia over thorax, abdomen and pubis extending laterally to the mid-axillary lines and infero-laterally into the groin (Fig. 103).

Subgroup 8: Stimulation from second web of the right forepaw to second web of left forepaw. An area of cutaneous anesthesia over thorax, abdomen, and pubis extending laterally to the midaxillary lines (Fig. 104).

Subgroup 9: Stimulation from second web of right forepaw to vertex. An area of cutaneous anesthesia over the thorax, abdomen and pubis with extension of anesthesia to the elbow and knee joints of the etxremities (Fig. 105).

Subgroup 10: Stimulation from vertex to second web of right forepaw.

Subgroup 11: Stimulation from vertex to second web of right hind paw. In subgroup 10 and 11 and area of cutaneous anesthesia over thorax and upper abdomen between nipple lines (Fig. 106).

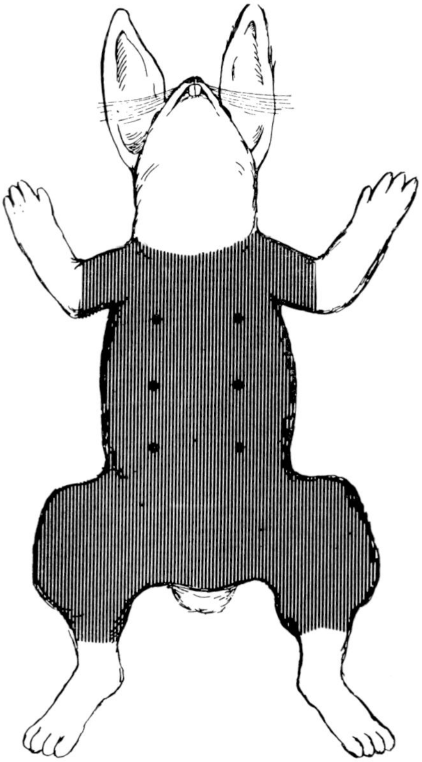

Figure 103: Area of local anesthesia following electric stimulation; "second web of right hind paw to vertex."

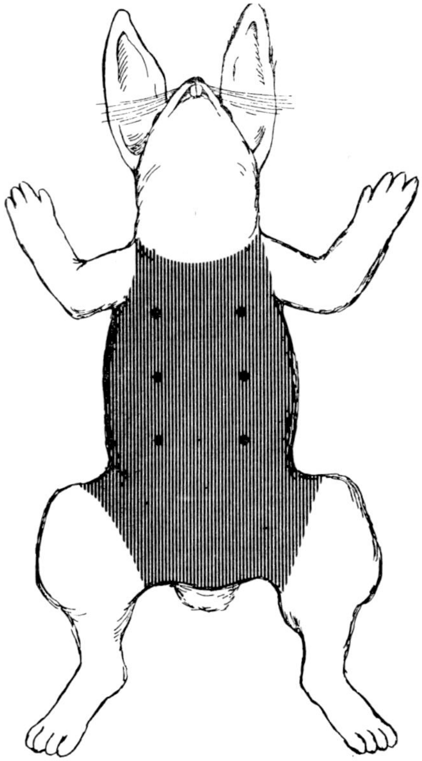

Figure 104: Area of local anesthesia following electric stimulation; second web of the right forepaw to second web of left forepaw."

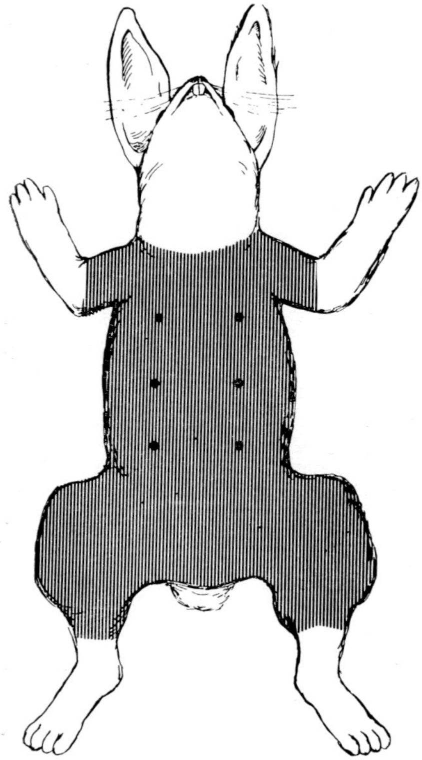

Figure 105: Area of local anesthesia following electric stimulation; "second web of right forepaw to vertex."

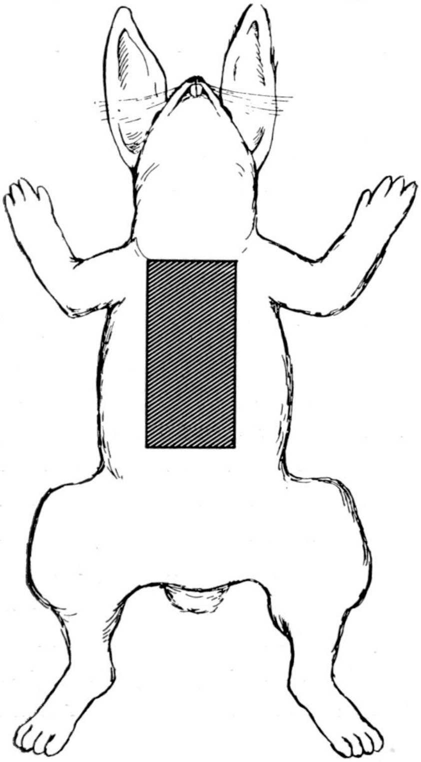

Figure 106: Area of local anesthesia following electric stimulation; "vertex to second web of right hind paw."

There was no change in blood pressure, pulse, ECG or eye signs in the animals studied either during or after electrical stimulation when compared to the pre-stimulation baseline tracings.

Discussion

It is important to know whether or not there are specific points which will produce acupuncture anesthesia.

The traditional acupuncture points have been selected on the basis of the meridian line and meridian point concepts.[77] Recently it has been shown in humans that meridian points correspond well to electrically sensitive points on the skin.[11]

Unfortunately, in the rabbit, there was no difference in electrical sensitivity at any point on its skin except for digital webs. This would seem to suggest that either the rabbit has no meridian lines or points, or more practically the animal has no cutaneous areas of decreased skin resistance even over the sites of superficial major peripheral nerves.

From our experimental data we have noted the following:

1. The Area of anesthesia starts centrally over the thorax and then spreads peripherally to the abdomen, axilla, groin and finally the extremities.
2. Anesthesia was present fifteen to thirty minutes after start of electrical stimulation.
3. Anesthesia was present forty-five minutes after onset of manual stimulation over the thorax and upper abdomen.
4. Electrical stimulation produced no change in BP, pulse, or ECG.
5. The direction of current was critical, since the best results were obtained in conducting the current from the second web of the forepaw to the vertex and from the second web of the hind paw to the vertex.
6. During all of the experiments the animals remained alert. There was no observation of roving eye movements. There were no pupillary changes and the animals always retained their blink response.

Any explanation of the pathophysiologic mechanism of acupuncture at this time is almost philosophical. According to the Gate Theory,[4] the stimulation of the large fibers entering the dorsal horn stimulates a regulator cell in the substantia gelatinosa which in turn blocks the transmission of pain impulses by a transmitter cell located in the dorsal horn. When the large fibers are not stimulated, pain impulses are conducted to this transmitter cell by the small non-myelinated fibers and these impulses are then conducted to the thalamus and cortex. It may be possible that, acupuncture acts as a stimulator of the large myelinated fibers which in turn stimulate the cell in the substantia gelatinosa and block the transmitter cell.[78] Recent work by Man and Citen postulate a second gate in the thalamus which they suggest has to do with regulation of facial pain.[79] Indeed, it is even possible that there are several gates located in the cord, brain stem and thalamus. The fact that the direction of current was critical in our study may indicate some relation to the existence of such a theory.

We do not feel that acupuncture anesthesia will offer an alternative to current modes of anesthesia. Rather we think that it will be another weapon in the anesthesiologist's armamentarium. Because of this we feel that more intensive study will be directed to this interesting concept recently introduced into western medicine.

Summary

Cutaneous anesthesia was produced in rabbits within minutes by manual or electric stimulation of acupuncture needles placed subcutaneously.

Efficacy of the anesthesia differed according to location(s) of the needle. No changes were produced in BP, pulse, ECG, or eye signs.

The area of anesthesia started centrally and spread gradually to the extremities. With electric stimulation, the direction of the electric current was critical and best results were obtained when electric current was introduced from the second web of the forepaw or hind paw to the vertex.

ACUPUNCTURE AND POST VAGOTOMY GASTROINTESTINAL ATONY

Recent reports from the Peoples' Republic of China regarding the value of acupuncture have given the public the impression that this is rather empirical and that one may treat it with skepticism. However, interest in acupuncture has been growing among physicians in this country. Acupuncture has been used for over 3,000 years to relieve pain and treat various physical disorders in China, but the concept of acupuncture anesthesia has only been introduced recently. This specific concept of utilizing acupuncture as anesthesia for surgery is what is attracting the attention of U. S. physicians.

Evaluation of acupuncture and acupuncture anesthesia has been continuing in this laboratory.[80] In our measurement of skin potential of normal and diseased patients, it was found that *meridian points* (acupuncture points) were areas where somatic nerves were located superficially and could easily be detected objectively by the use of a galvanic device. In addition, in the disease patient skin potential at these meridian points, which is said to be specifically related to the particular disorder, revealed changing electric permeability compared to that in other meridian points on the same patient.

A by-product of this study was recognition of the fact that electric permeability was reduced in certain gastric meridian points following vagotomy.

The objective of this study then was to evaluate the efficacy of acupuncture in the management of gastrointestinal atony following vagotomy.

Materials and Methods

A total of twenty-four adult white rabbits of both sexes were used for this study. It was essential to prepare the bowel for five days prior to surgery since multiple small fecal balls filled the rectum and these fecal balls fell out easily with minimum physical movement. Rabbits were clipped and depilated with Nair® cream, four hours prior to the experiment. Rabbits were divided equally into four groups according to the procedure to be carried out on them. All animals were immobilized on the operating table in a supine position, and anesthetized with ether by open drop technique.

In the first group of six animals, laparotomy through a midline incision originating in the subxyphoid area was made and the peritoneum was entered. The stomach was retracted inferiorly and the esophagogastric junction was freed from surrounding tissue. An umbilical tape was placed around the esophagus, then removed. No vagus nerves were severed. The wound was closed in a standard manner. In the second, third and fourth group of six animals each, complete bilateral truncal vagotomy was performed using a similar incision and maneuvers to those used in the animals in the first group. The wound was closed in a standard manner in each animal.

In each rabbit in Groups 2, 3, and 4, the electric permeability was measured at various areas on the entire body surface. Acupuncture with

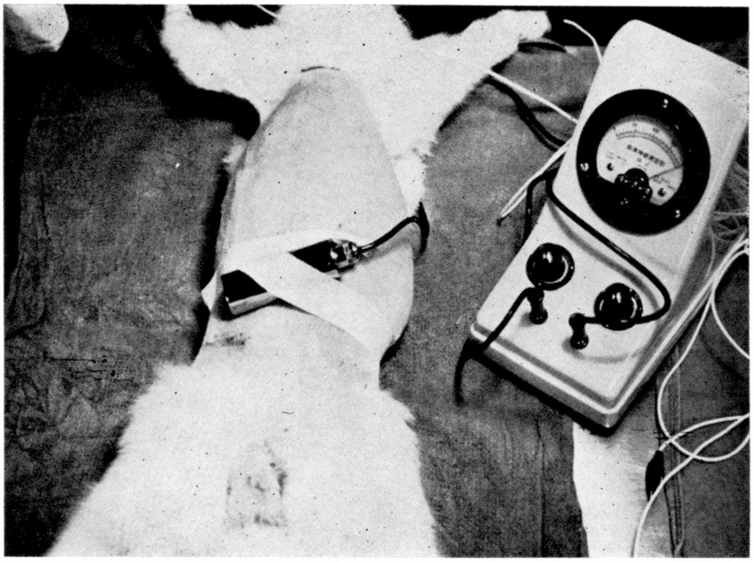

Figure 107: Dispensive electrode of the neurometer is now attached to the rabbit's abdomen (note the hair has been removed).

electric stimulation was applied at the gluteal meridian point where decreased electric permeability was noted. It was applied on the third day after vagotomy in the third group of six animals and immediately after vagotomy in the six animals in the fourth group.

Measurement of electrically permeable points was done with a Neurometer, a galvanic device. An L-C type neurometer was used for this study. Meter reading was adjusted at 200 microamperes (uA) after the detecting electrode and the dispensive electrode had been shunted together across 12 volts on the device (Fig. 4). The dispensive electrode was attached to the animal's lower abdomen (Fig. 107). The detecting electrode was held by an examiner, and its point was placed at various areas over the entire skin surface, and a meter reading was obtained at each point. A meter reading of less than 200 uA indicated decreased electric permeability and, conversely, increased skin resistance at a particular point.

As was stated acupuncture was given at a point in the gluteal area after confirming a change in measurement of electric permeability of the point by using the neurometer. A No. 3 acupuncture needle (diameter of needle was 0.24 mm) (Fig. 8) was inserted 1 cm in depth at this point. Electric stimulation was then supplied by the neurometer by attaching the dis-

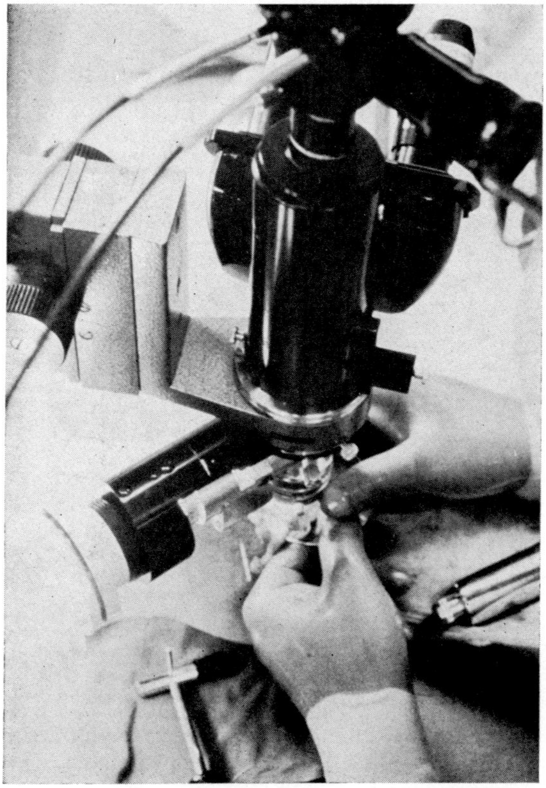

Figure 108: Intravital microscopy.

pensive electrode to the acupuncture needle at a dial setting of 12 volts and 200 uA for thirty minutes.

Bowel sounds were checked twice daily and the day of initial defecation after surgery was recorded. An ultropak intravital microscope was used to evaluate microcirculation of the mesentery through a small laparotomy three days after vagotomy (Fig. 108).

Results

In all acupuncture points on each animal's skin, the reading on the neurometer was 170 uA at the various points evaluated before surgery.

The readings in animals in which no vagotomy was performed (Group 1) revealed no changes at any point on the body after laparotomy up to ten days postoperatively, while in animals in which vagotomy was performed (Group 2), the reading reduced gradually to 160, 150 and 130 uA at their shoulder and the gluteal area at one, two, and three days after surgery. Readings remained between 130 to 140 uA for the next seven days. However, in animals in which acupuncture with electric stimulation was given at three days after surgery, at which time the reading was 130 uA (Group 3), the reading returned to 140, 150, and 165 uA fifth, sixth, and seventh post-vagotomy day but never returned to 170 uA over the next three days (Fig. 109).

Time required for return of bowel sounds following vagotomy was an average two days in the group where acupuncture with electric stimulation was given (Group 3) and three days in the group where no acupuncture

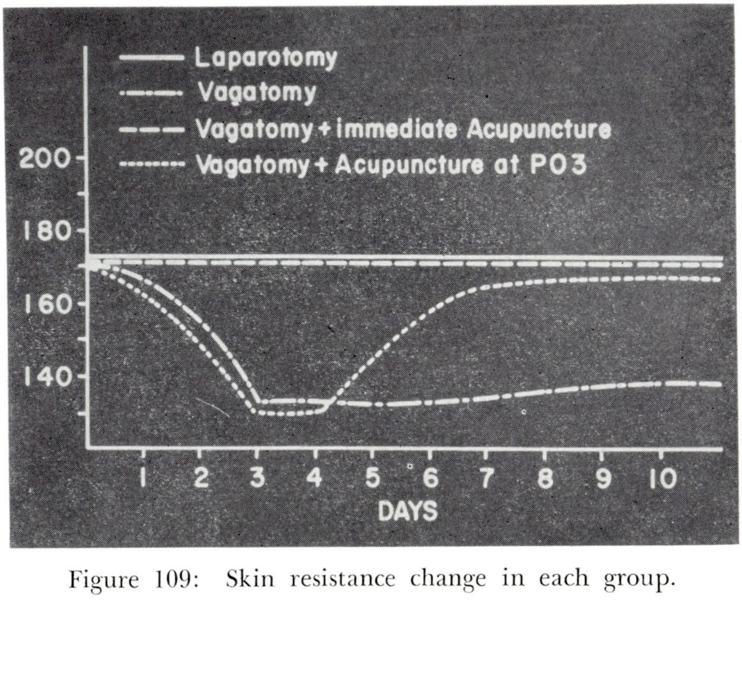

Figure 109: Skin resistance change in each group.

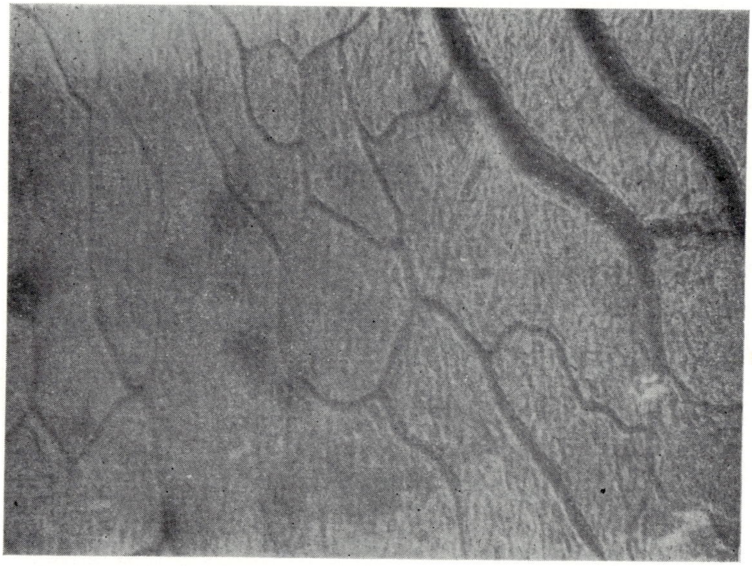

Figure 110: Microcirculation in Group 3.

was given (Group 2). Time required for the initial bowel movement was one to two days in the former group while it was two to four days in the latter group.

Intravital microscope study indicated minimum aggregation in venules with active flow in the third group (Fig. 110) while it revealed constricted vasculature and aggregation with minimum flow in the second group (Fig. 111).

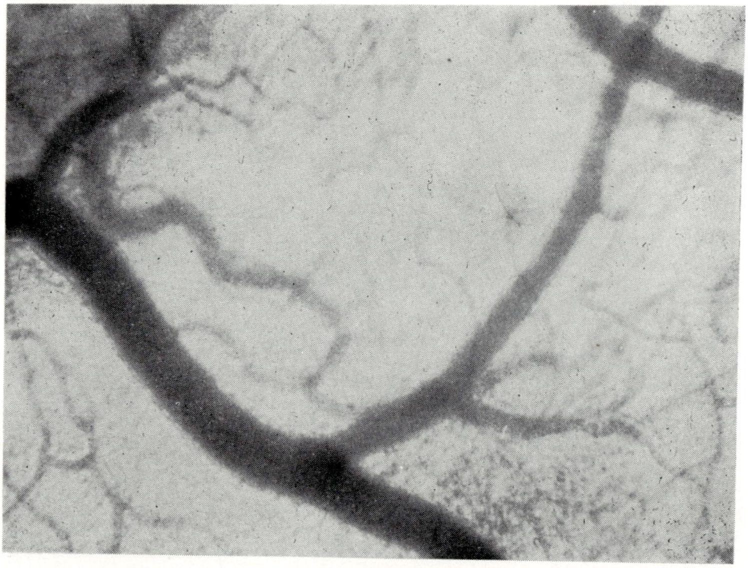

Figure 111: Microcirculation in Group 4.

Comment

Truncal vagotomy has been known to reduce gastric tone and prolong gastric emptying time. Vagotomy disrupts the gastric pacemaker potentials for approximately five days.[81] Multiple pacemakers arise in the stomach following vagotomy and propagate pacemaker potentials in various directions. Thus, uncoordinated gastric contraction accounts for the gastric stasis.

Recovery from the altered electrical pattern takes place approximately one week after vagotomy. However, the velocity of propagation of the gastric pacesetter potential through the gastric wall remains slowed permanently.[81,82] Other causes of delayed gastric emptying after vagotomy are due to the fact that vagotomy abolishes vagal release of gastrin and diminishes gastric contraction by Insulin and fats.[81,82] Thus, the motor changes after vagotomy are believed to be the consequence of changes in the pattern of gastroelectrical activity caused by the surgery.

The observation and analysis of Chinese physicians over long periods of time of the effects on signs and symptoms, following irritation of varying degrees at certain points on the body surface, made it possible to relate the most effective points on the body to the cure of some specific disorders. These points were named meridian points.

According to the ancient Chinese clinical concepts, the meridian points served as *peeping holes* into the body, and *passing holes* for energy. Each was named by its effect, anatomical location, appearance and relation to the meridian line. These meridian points were selected initially according to measurements based on the patient's own unique anatomical standard (using the length between certain anatomical points, for example, between nipples). The exact location of a meridian point is then selected by the examiner who feels with his finger tips the area chosen by the initial measurement and watches the patient's response.

However, these points are best elucidated by use of a neurometer to define the resistive areas electrically. Anatomically, some of the meridian points seem to correspond to an area where a nerve appears to surface from a muscle or an area where vessels and nerves are located relatively superficially, such as in areas between a muscle and a bone, a bone and a joint, etc.

To date, there is no ideal technique to measure autonomic activity. Metabolic determinations by the gasometric or by gas analysis method are not only difficult to obtain but are of questionable validity. Neurophysiologic investigation indicates that measurement of electric phenomenon of the skin provides an index of activity of the sympathetic nervous system.[83] Study indicated skin resistance varies with location of the skin area and the technique of measurement.[84,85] In this study, a galvanic device which has been routinely used by Japanese acupuncturists was used to determine a relative value and therefore the results presented here are not absolute values of skin resistance. This simple galvanic device provides the capability of specifying the relative value of skin resistance instantaneously. Due to the poor response to a galvanic device of rabbit's skin, specific study in relation to the various meridian points and gastropathophysiology is now being studied in the primate. The poor galvanic response of rabbit's skin may possibly be due to a lack of sweat glands on the body surface.

A distinct difference in skin resistance, however, before, and after vagotomy was significant and noted in all animals. This fact, also, presents the hypothesis that measurement of skin resistance may provide an index of completeness of vagotomy in a relatively simple fashion. Acupuncture with electric stimulation was advantageously used to maintain preoperative skin resistance. In addition, acupuncture with electric stimulation definitely improved post vagotomy gastrointestinal atony. From our study, it is thought that there is some relationship between autonomic nervous system function in the stomach and electric stimulation on the meridian points. It is necessary to repeat the same experiment in primates who have different sweat gland activities on body surface due to sympathetic regulation. It is speculated, however, that in primates the specific location of the meridian point where the acupuncture needle with electric stimulation should be applied would be detected easily by measuring changes in skin resistance following vagotomy. In humans, whether or not the point which reveals maximum reduction in skin resistance following vagotomy is located on the Chinese traditional gastric meridian is now being evaluated.

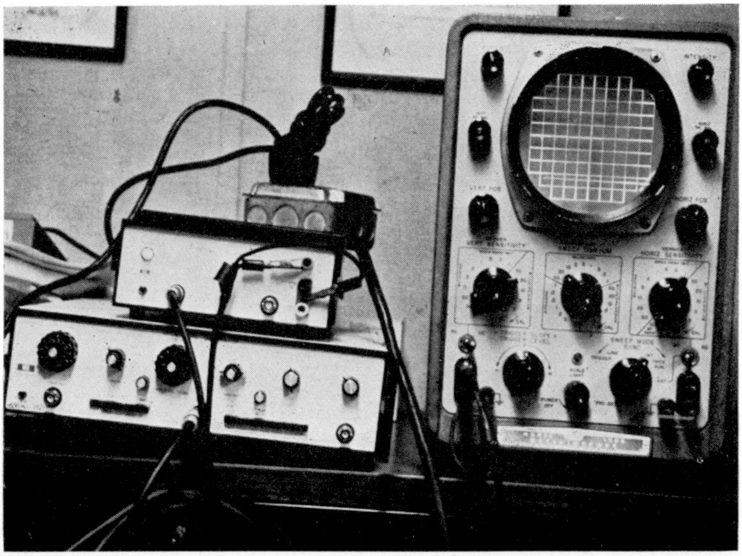

Figure 112: Electrical devices provide different voltage, cycle and wave shape with ossilograph.

The type of electric current (A.C., D.C.), cycle, voltage, pulse interval and wave shape (Fig. 112) to be applied from the acupuncture needle must also be evaluated to obtain the best results. Electric stimulation on the meridian point may improve the altered gastric pacemaker potential promptly.

Summary

Skin resistance changed significantly at the meridian point following vagotomy in rabbits. Application of an acupuncture needle with electric stimulation on the meridian point minimizes change of skin resistance. Reduction of gastrointestinal motility following vagotomy is also minimized by this application.

The animal's foreleg was dissected and each tissue was exposed. Stimulation of each tissue was provided by acupuncture with or without electric current. In our limited study, stimulation of muscles and tenons did not cause anesthesia while stimulation of nerve tissues did. The best results were obtained when radial nerve was stimulated.

Degree of analgesia was tested in humans while first dorsal web (gokoku, hoku) was stimulated manually. Continuous EEG was obtained (Figs. 113-117). However, it is essential to use more sophisticated equipment and to evaluate sensory evoked potential in order to obtain meaningful data.

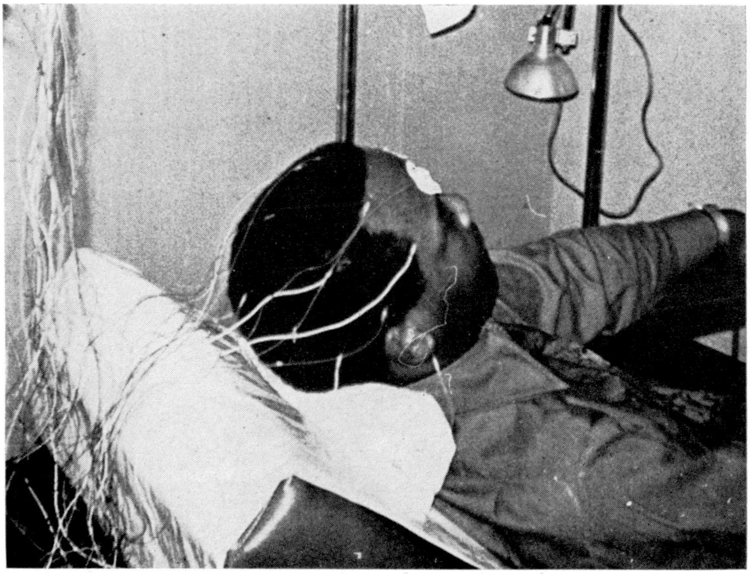

Figure 113: EEG electrodes are placed.

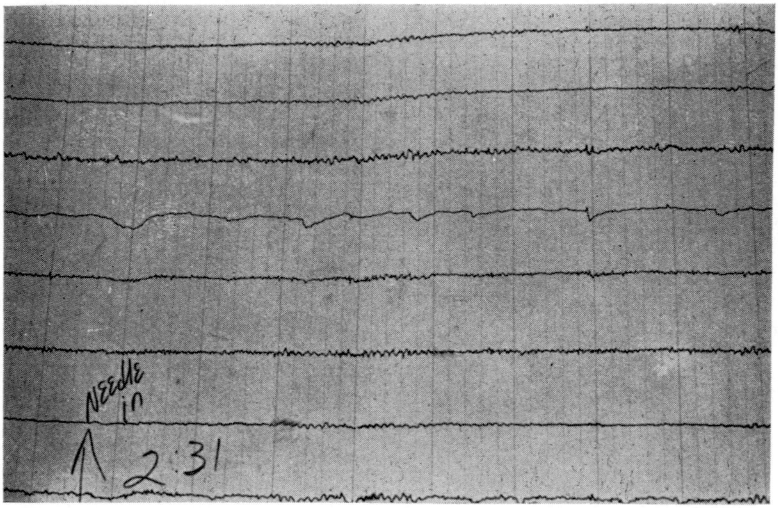

Figure 114: EEG finding: an acupuncture needle is placed in left first dorsal web (gokoku, hoku) and twirling is started.

CLINICAL EVALUATION OF ACUPUNCTURE IN CHRONIC NECK AND SHOULDER PAIN DUE TO OSTEOARTHRITIS

Acupuncture has been used for more than 2,000 years in China and Far Eastern countries with considerable acceptance.[14,42,87] In this long period, no known serious complications have been reported with its use. In the United States, however, acupuncture has been greeted with a great deal of skepticism because of the lack of scientific explanations and objective

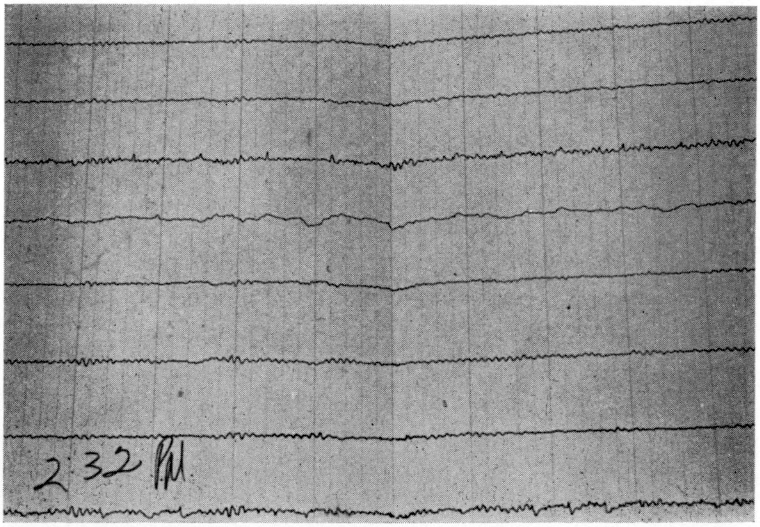

Figure 115: EEG finding: one minute later after insertion of the needle.

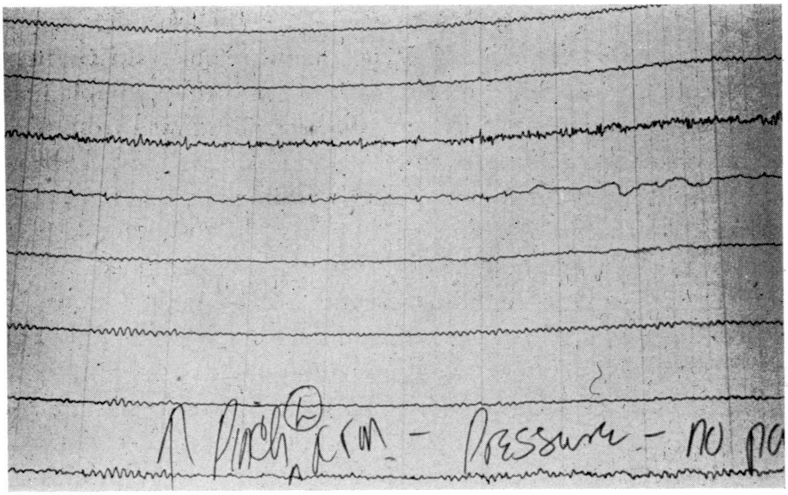

Figure 116: EEG finding: left elbow, shoulder and neck are compressed and pinched with tweezer. No pain is felt.

studies regarding its use. Experimental animal studies of acupuncture and acupuncture anesthesia done in this laboratory for the past year have been previously reported.[80,87]

The purpose of this chapter is to report clinical experience with acupuncture used as treatment for patients with chronic neck pain due to osteoarthritis.

Methods of Procedure

A. Patients:

A total of twenty-four reliable adults of both sexes ranging in age from

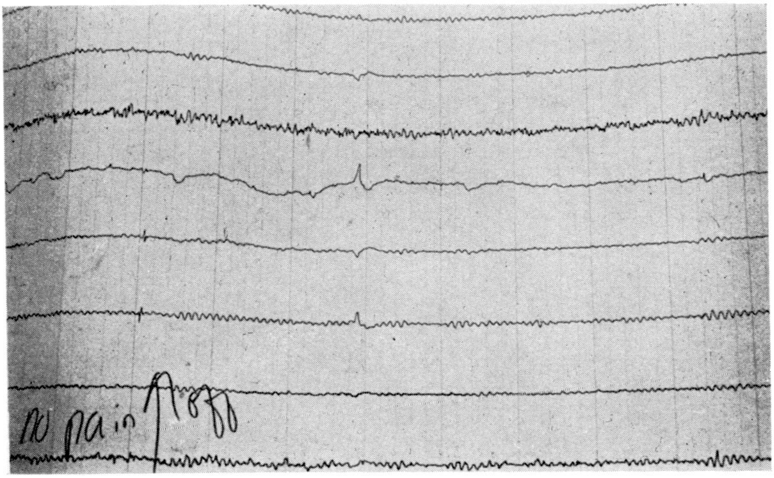

Figure 117: No pain is felt with Kocher clamping of arm and shoulder.

forty-five to fifty-five years and with complaints of shoulder pain due to cervical osteoarthritis were studied. Other than the osteoarthritis, none were acutely ill. Patients with mental instability or multiple complaints which were not related to their specific diagnosis were eliminated from this study. Patients included housewives, businessmen, physicians, and salesmen. All were screened carefully for indications as well as to ensure nonexistence of other diseases which could cause similar pain. In this study, patients with herniated discs or who had had previous surgery were excluded.

Diagnostic procedures including careful history taking, range of neck motion, reliable x-rays of cervical spine and shoulder joints (myelogram in some patients) and laboratory work up (CBC, urinalysis, SMA-12, PTT, and uric acid) had been completed in all patients within six months prior to the acupuncture treatments. If any of the previous studies were not completed within a prior six month period, additional work-ups, as needed, were completed before beginning treatment. All patients had no other positive physical findings with the exception of osteoarthritis of the cervical spine. They all had been treated by rheumatologist, neurosurgeons and/or orthopedic surgeons, in addition to their family physicians for more than one year without appreciable improvement and were referred by one of these physicians.

Patients were requested to sign a permit prior to acupuncture after being given a careful explanation of the procedure. No acupuncture was given on the initial visit but rather efforts were made not only to screen the patients to be sure they would meet study criteria but also to obtain their full understanding of the procedures and the importance of their assistance in obtaining accurate data. Evaluation of mental stability was also made.

B. Grouping and Technique:

Twenty-four patients were divided into two groups (equally) according to the method of stimulation. Group 1 received manual needle stimulation and Group 2 received electric needle stimulation.

In the patients of Group 1, the method of control was by single blind study. A traditional acupuncture point coinciding with the most tender point of the neck and shoulder which also had significantly altered electric activity of skin was selected. An acupuncture needle was introduced 1 cm in depth perpendicular to the skin and advanced in various directions until the patient felt an aching, radiating distally or proximally (so-called *Needle Feeling*).

Two other points which were not tender, not on the traditional acapuncture point or meridian line and revealed no altered electric activity of the skin were selected and a needle was inserted in each to the same depth (Fig. 118). The fact that the patient did not experience the *Needle Feeling* was confirmed at these two points.

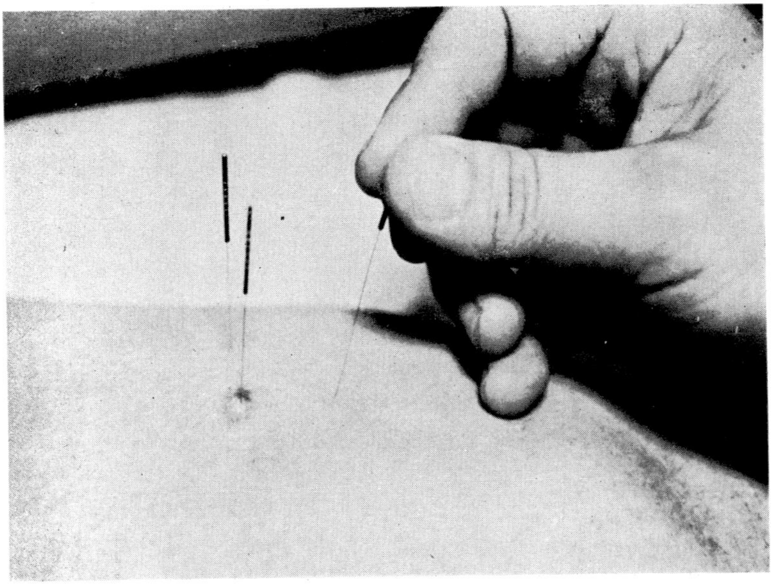

Figure 118: Needles were inserted into the acupuncture point and two control points.

The galvanic device used in this study was a L-C type neurometer (Fig. 4). Meter reading was adjusted to 200 microamperes with the dispensive electrode being gently held in the patient's left hand with a constant pressure. The detecting electrode was held by an examiner. Its point was placed on various areas of the skin surface with a constant pressure and a meter reading of more than 100 units was defined as the point with increased electric sensitivity.

Patients in Group 1, a total of twelve, were divided into three subgroups:

Subgroup 1 (4 patients): *Sparrow pecking* and twirling motion at the specific point were alternated every minute for ten minutes.

Subgroup 2 (4 patients): *Sparrow pecking* and twirling motion of the needle on the control points were alternated every minute for ten minutes.

Subgroup 3 (4 patients): No motion applied to needle. Needle located at another control point.

In the patients of Group 2, the three needles were placed by a physician but each electric lead was attached to each needle by a third person. The device was so arranged that one of the leads was connected to the battery and was live, another lead was connected to the battery but was not live, and the last lead was not even connected to the battery at all. These connections were not identifiable from outside by anyone. Thus, patient and evaluating physician did not know which needle was in the specific point and which lead was actually introducing the electric current (double-blind study) (Fig 119).

Patients in Group 2, a total of twelve patients, were subdivided into three groups:

Subgroup 1 (4 patients): 200 mA of electric current were applied at the specific point for five minutes and no current was applied to two other control points.

Subgroup 2 (4 patients): 200 mA of electric current were applied to one of the control points for five minutes and no current was given to the specific and other control points.

Subgroup 3 (4 patients): 200 mA of electric current were applied to another control point for five minutes and no current was given to the specific and other control points.

Each patient was questioned immediately after removal of the needles as to improvement in terms of less pain or more motion. The same procedure was repeated every seventy-two hours, from three to ten individual visits. In all patients, points where a needle was inserted were recorded and marked accurately at each visit so the original points could be identified and reused. Efficacy was determined by degree of pain and motion described on a scale both before and after the procedure at each visit following the

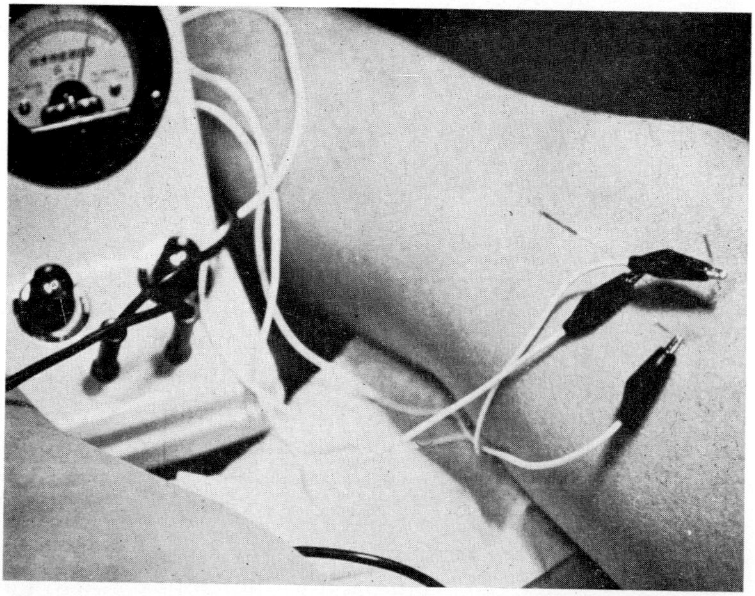

Figure 119: Needles were inserted into the acupuncture point and two other control points. One needle was connected to the battery and two others were not.

second visit. Studies were done of pre and post treatment activity and performance levels and pain tolerances. Samples were taken of daily activity schedules in relation to reported pain status. Dosage, frequency and type of analgesics taken by patients were carefully checked and compared to that taken both pre and post acupuncture therapy. These patients were also trained to compare the effect of acupuncture with other previous therapies. On successive visits, if pain disappeared and skin sensitivity decreased to the normal level at some of the points where acupuncture had been given, no further treatment was given at these points.

Results

Approximately 80 percent of the traditional Chinese acupuncture points revealed altered electric activity of the skin (increased sensitivity) and these points were always tender by finger pressure[6]. All patients did not feel definite *Needle Feeling* unless the needle was placed in the traditional acupuncture points.

After the initial treatment, all patients in Subgroup 1 of both groups (those who received manual needle motion or 200 mA of electric current at the specific point) noted immediate improvement of pain after treatment. They were able to move their neck and shoulder more extensively without pain compared to pretreatment status.

After each visit, the patients in these subgroups felt further improvement and required less frequent and less potent medication. They noted more activity and more motion of the neck, except for one patient in Group 1, Subgroup 1 and one patient in Group 2, Subgroup 1, who had temporary increase of pain the night of the initial treatment. Two patients in Group 1, Subgroup 1 and one patient in Group 2, Subgroup 1 were discharged after three treatments with satisfactory recovery. Each of the remaining five patients in Subgroup 1 of Groups 1 and 2 except one in Group 2 improved at each visit continuously but none completely after four to ten visits. The patient is Subgroup 1 of Group 2 improved after each treatment but the improvement remained for less than forty-eight hours. The improved condition in these patients was maintained from three to seven months with one series of treatment. One patient in Group 2, Subgroup 1 required three treatments, with excellent response at each visit, every two months for a six month period.

Of all the patients in Subgroups 2 and 3 of Groups 1 and 2, no one experienced continuous improvement for more than three days. All the other patients in the control groups noted no improvement at all, after both initial and successive treatments. Four patients in these subgroups noted improvement for twenty-four to forty-eight hours after the first and second treatment only. No further improvement was noted.

TABLE V

Results of Acupuncture Controlled Study

Group	Subgroup	Patient Number	Serial of Treatment 1	2	3	4	5	6	7	8	9	10
1	1	1	+	++	++	++	++	++	++	++		
		2	+	++	++	Discharged						
		3	+	−+	−+	++	++	++	++			
		4	+	++	++	Discharged						
	2	1	−	−+	−−	−+	−+	++	++	−		
		2	±	−−	−−	−+	++	++	Discharged			
		3	−	−−	−−	−−	++	++	++	Discharged		
		4	−	−+	−−	−+	−+	−+	−+	++	++	
	3	1	−	−	−	−	−	−	−	−	−	
		2	−	−	−	−	−					
		3	−	−	−	−	−					
		4	−	−	−	−	−					
2	1	1	+	++	++	Discharged						
		2	+	++	++	++	++	++	++	++	++	++
		3	+	−+	−+	−+	−+	−+	++	++		
		4	+	−−	−−	−+	−+	−+	−+	−+	−+	−+
	2	1	+	+−	−−	−+	++	++	++	Discharged		
		2	−	−−	−−	−+	−+	−−	Discharged			
		3	−	−−	−−	−−	−−	−+	−+	−+	−+	Dis-charged
		4	−	−−	−−	−−	−+	++	++	−+	−+	−+
	3	1	−	−−	−−	−+	−+	−+	−+	−+		
		2	−	−−	−−	−+	++	++	Discharged			
		3	−	−+	−−	−−	−−	−+	−+	−+	−+	−+
		4	−	−−	−−	−−	−+	++	++	Discharged		

Each patient in Subgroups 2 and 3 of Groups 1 and 2 received the stimulation at the specific point following three successive treatments without appreciable improvement. The results were tabulated in Table V.

Discussion

Despite a vast literature concerning acupuncture, an objective study of acupuncture has not yet been reported. Oriental reports leave one impressed with the efficacy of acupuncture for the various ailments but again, reports of the objective study are lacking.

On the other hand, public demand for acupuncture has been growing while the AMA's stand regarding the practice of acupuncture is neither approval or disapproval. It is therefore absolutely necessary to clarify efficacy in a scientific manner. Scientific speculation among physicians has been reported. Doctor Kroger[88] in a letter to the Editor (JAMA) pointed out that acupuncture is a form of hypnosis, while others believe the efficacy of acupuncture could be explained by concept of Gate Control Theory or its modification speculating the existence of multiple gates.

In any event, it is essential to know whether acupuncture is effective for certain conditions and if it is whether stimulation should be given at the specific points or whether any point on the body will be effective. Since the anatomical location of the acupuncture points described in traditional texts are numerous and not precise, a galvanic device was added to pinpoint the location rather than using numerous acupuncture points which also had altered electric activity of the skin. When manual stimulation is used, double blind study is impossible; but by placing three needles, the patient does not realize which is being stimulated. In addition, almost all patients have a preconceived idea that acupuncture is painless. They are unaware of the necessity of *Needle Feeling* during the procedure. Thus, the patient does not know if the correct acupuncture point is being stimulated.

When electric current was used, a double blind study was undertaken. For the same reasons described above, the patients in these subgroups of Group 2 did not know which point was being stimulated. Since the physician only placed the needle in each point and the technician only attached a wire from a battery box and only one wire was alive, neither physician nor patient, nor technician were aware of which point was being stimulated with the electric current. Thus this part of the experiment could be considered a double blind study.

Our study indicates that 70 percent of the traditional acupuncture points are actually points where electric activity of the skin is significantly altered. It is speculated that these points were those where somatic nerve branches run relatively superficially. It is necessary, however, to evaluate efficacy of acupuncture given at traditional acupuncture points but where the electric activity of the skin is unaltered. Japanese investigators[12] accept the points where electric activity of the skin is altered as acupuncture points and name them as *Ryodo Ketsu* (electrically permeable hall).

This study indicates that the stimulation must be given to specific points. When the stimulation was given on nonspecific points, the patient noticed improvement of pain only on some occasions. However, there is a statistically significant difference noted concerning the success rate between cases in which stimulation was given to specific as opposed to nonspecific points. Although there is no statistical difference, it was our impression that manual stimulation is more effective compared to stimulation with electric current. This may be due to the fact that manual manipulation can alter the degree of stimulation at each treatment while the electric current given in this study was more or less a constant stimulus.

The mechanism of action of acupuncture is not understood at this time. Traditional explanations of the five element theory and positive and negative forces concept prevented scientific explanation for a long period of time. At present, explanations of the mechanisms of acupuncture are speculative and based on physiological, particularly neurophysiological data. Some consider acupuncture a mode of hypnosis. However, the fact that acupuncture does work in animals has been shown in our laboratory[80,87]. In addition, our clinical experiments mitigate against this concept. In our study, application of the needle apart from the specific meridian points proved to be of no value. Its application on the specific points was effective. In this regard, we have been inclined to believe that efficacy of acupuncture is primarily due to neurophysiologic mechanisms rather than hypnotic action.

Modern medicine as developed in the western hemisphere and now practiced throughout the world appears to be highly effective in the cure of disease. However, there are still certain syndromes and diseases for which modern medicine is not indicated or even effective. Chronic pain is certainly one of them and frequently becomes a problem for the patient himself, then the family and even the nation. The patients suffering from chronic pain due to osteoarthritis are considerable in number and may be helped by properly conducted acupuncture. It is essential, yet, that these patients be thoroughly evaluated medically in order not to lose the golden period during which an underlying disorder could possibly be treated effectively by standard modern medical therapy.

Summary

Single and double blind study of efficacy of acupuncture in treatment of chronic neck and shoulder pain due to osteoarthritis were performed. The study indicated that the acupuncture was effective and there was a statistically significant difference of the efficacy between the patient who received acupuncture at the specific point and non-specific point.

COMPARISON OF ACUPUNCTURE AND REGIONAL NERVE BLOCK POINTS

The advancement of knowledge and the increased popularity of general anesthesia has limited the application of regional anesthesia. However, this technique of regional anesthesia has been successfully used for patients with intractable pain at the Pain Study Center, Department of Surgery, Hahnemann Medical College and Hospital.

While in local anesthesia the anesthetic agent is injected into or around the nerve trunks leading to the painful area; in regional block anesthesia, the nerve trunk is injected with a local anesthetic at some point after it leaves the spinal cord. Success of this technique involves manual skill, but it also depends on a very detailed knowledge of the course of the nerves from the spinal cord to the various parts of the body. A needle is introduced through the skin and muscle layer to the nerve trunk into which it is desired to inject the local anesthetic. If the injection is successful, the area of the body supplied by the nerve trunk becomes insensitive within a few minutes.

Para vertebral block anesthesia and sacral block are also considered variants of the regional anesthesia. In the para vertebral block the nerves are blocked as they leave the vertebral foramina. These nerve blocks are given to prevent pain during an operation on the chest, abdomen and pelvis and also to relieve pain due to diseases in these locations.

Selection of the needle points for nerve blocks is determined by the simplicity and easiness of finding the location. On many occasions, the point is located where the nerve runs superficially and between or near a distinctly located anatomical landmark.

Despite the lack of objective study of acupuncture, the selection of meridian points has been described in detail. With over 3,000 years experience, each meridian point has been selected for various kinds of ailments[1]. However, when selecting the meridian points for the specific pain, it became clear that many of the meridian points are closely related or in some situations, identical to the point for nerve block of the similar pain.

Acupuncture based on long experience, and nerve block which developed based on the objective scientific explanation are both helpful for relieving pain and the points where placing the needles are surprisingly similar. If one believes the systemic effect of acupuncture given to the specific meridian points, nerve block on the similar points may not only provide a temporary pain relief but also the unknown systemic effects.

In other words, needles given on the nerve blocking point on the meridian line may act as a kind of stressor to the organ over which a meridian line passes.

Accordingly in this chapter some of the nerve blocking and acupuncture points which are identically located points are selected and compared for their effects (Table VI).

TABLE VI

Objectives of Various Nerve Block

BLOCK	OBJECTIVE
Cervical Epidural Block	Circulatory insufficiency and pain in neck, arm and upper chest.
Thoracic Epidural Block	Circulatory insufficiency and pain in neck, arm and upper chest.
Lumbar Epidural Block	Circulatory insufficiency and pain below abdominal level, back and leg aches.
Thoracic Sympathetic Block	
Upper Thoracic	Angina, arrythmia, asthma, pulmonary emboli, cardiospasm.
Lower Thoracic	Cholelithiasis (colic), gastric pain, renal stone (colic), pancreatic pain, paralytic ileus, hypertension.
Lumbar Sympathetic Block	Raynaud's disease, peripheral vascular disease of the leg.
Thoracic Somatic Nerve Block	Chest pain, herpes zoster, pain due to fracture of rib or sternum, intercostal neuralgia.
Lumbar Somatic Nerve Block	Pain due to fracture of spine, lower abdominal pain, inguinal pain, backache, anterior thigh pain.
Celiac Plexus Block	Intra-abdominal pain, cardiospasm, peptic ulcer, paralytic ileus, hypertension.
Trans-sacral Nerve Block	Sciatica, pain due to intrapelvic malignancy.

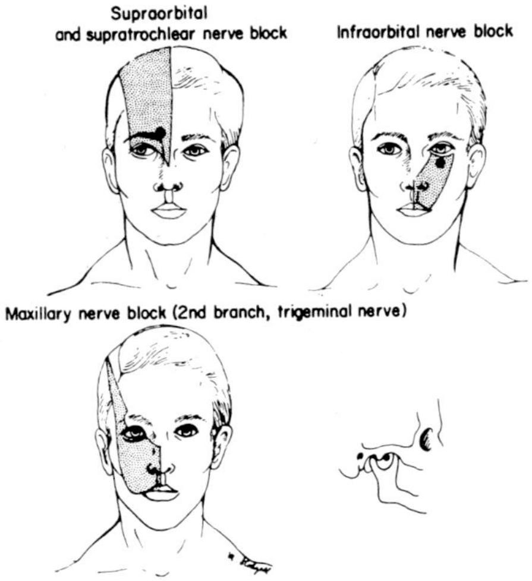

Figure 120: Median eyebrow, infraorbital, infratemporal.

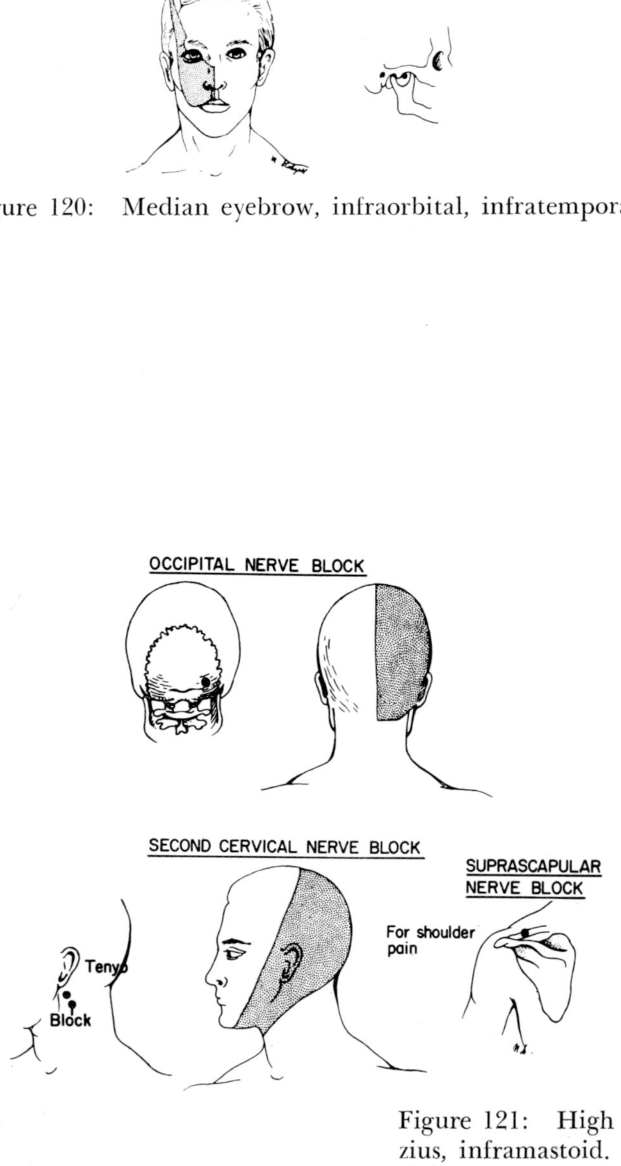

Figure 121: High lateral trapezius, inframastoid.

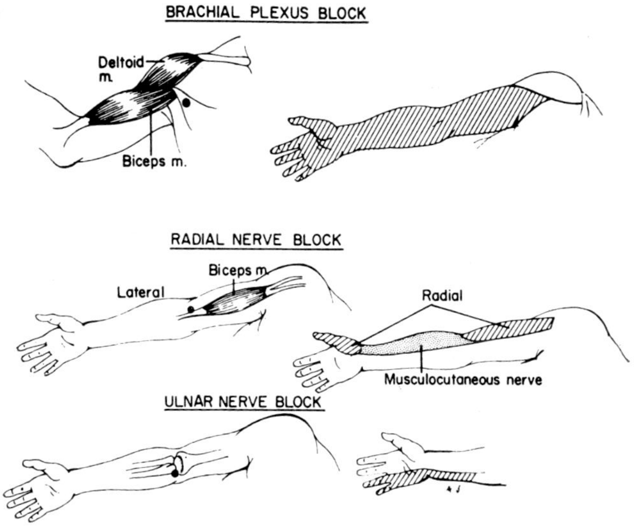

Figure 122: Axilla, radial antecubital, ulnar antecubital.

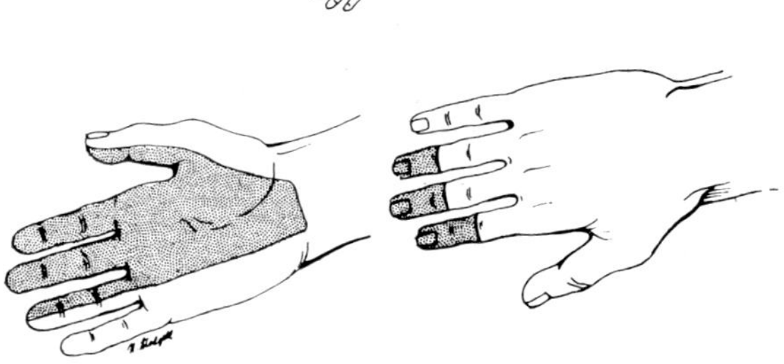

Figure 123: Antecubital.

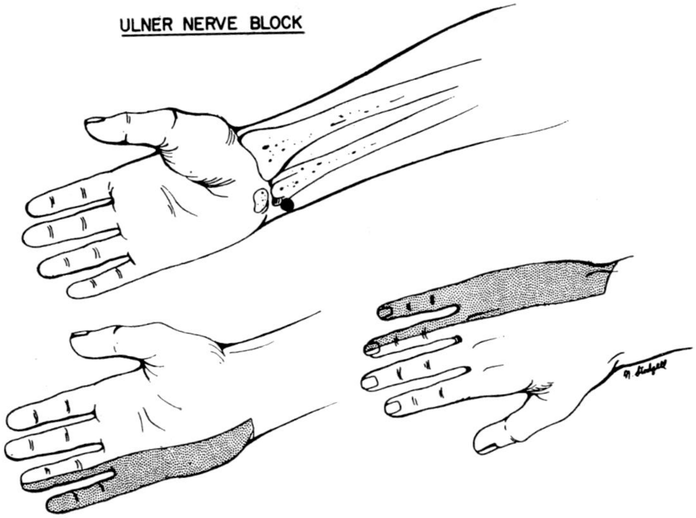

Figure 124: Ulnar volar wrist.

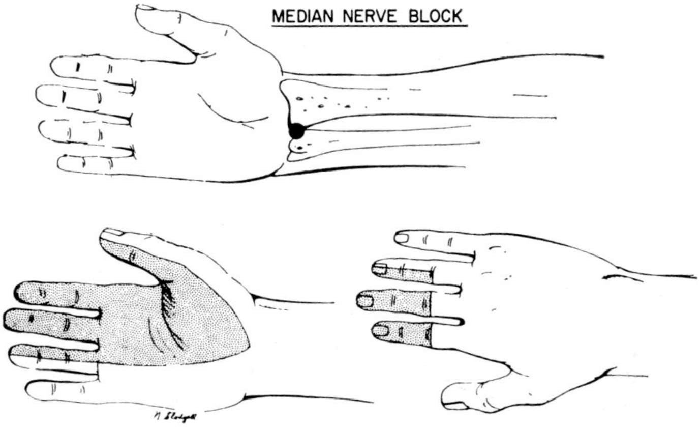

Figure 125: Midvolar wrist.

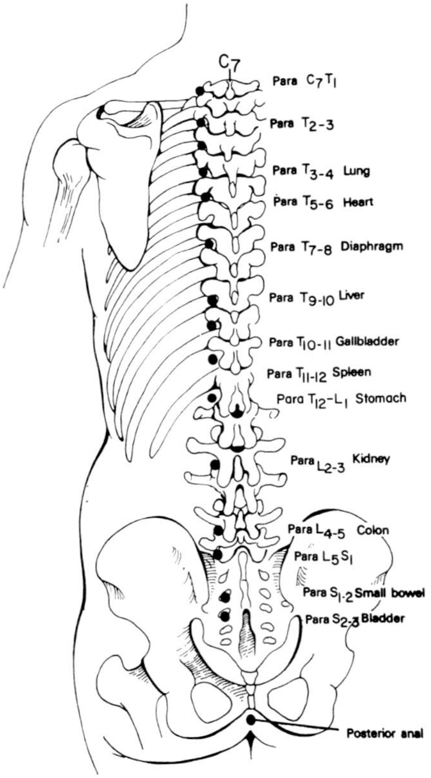

Figure 126: C7—T1, T1—T2, L2—L3, para T3—T4, para T5—T6, para T7—T8, para T9—T10, para T10—T11, para T11—T12, para T12—L1, para L2—L3, para L3—L4, lateral L2—L3.

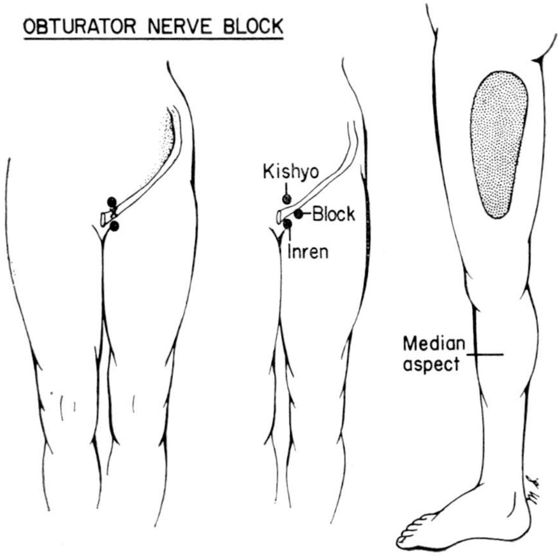

Figure 127: Median femoral.

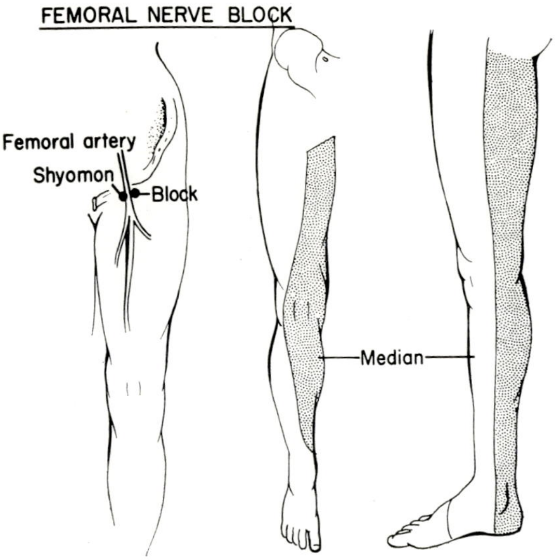

Figure 128: Femoral.

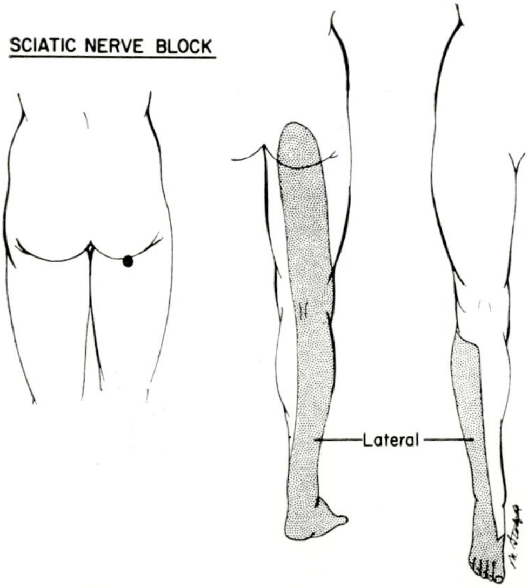

Figure 129: Midgluteal fold.

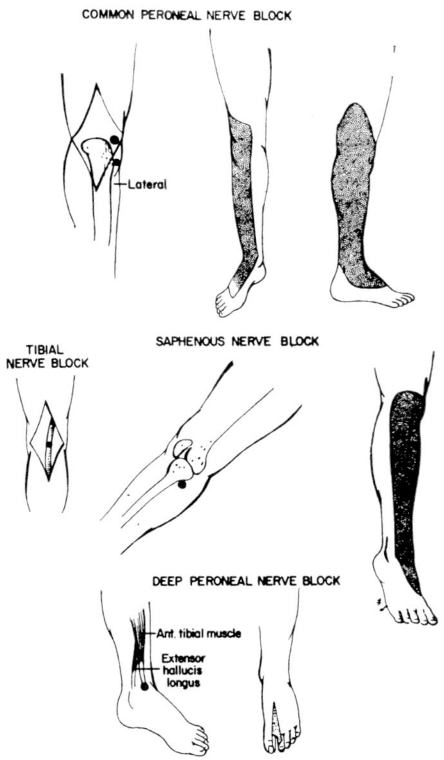

Figure 130: Anterior upper fibula, posterior upper tibia, anterior median ankle.

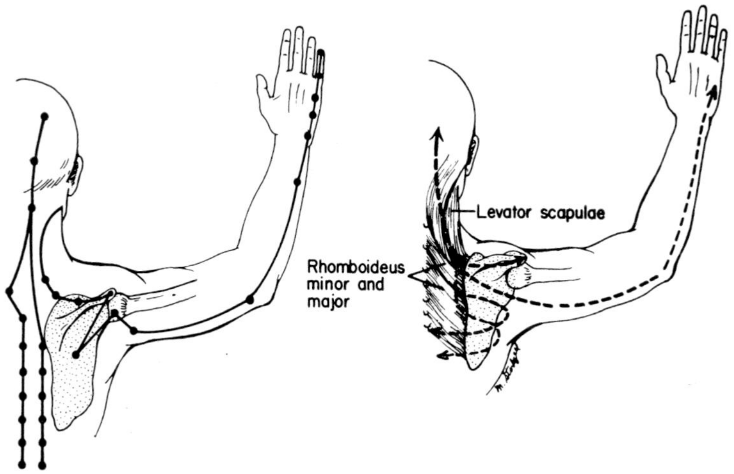

Figure 131: Direction of pain radiation.

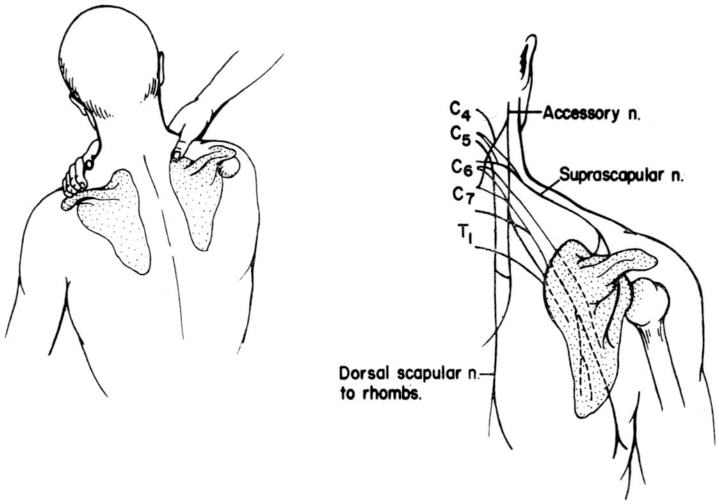

Figure 132: Scapulo costal syndrome; method of examination and nerve supply.

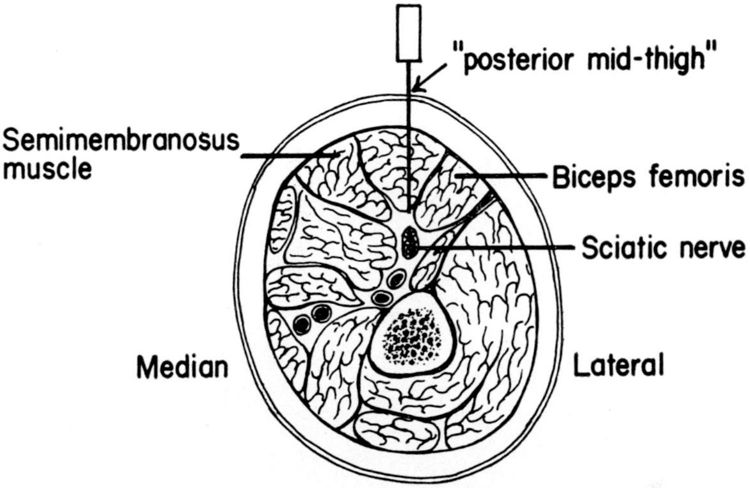

Figure 133: Relation of "posterior mid-thigh" point and sciatic nerve.

Meridian Point *(English)* *(Japanese)* *(Chinese)*	*Effect*	*Nerve Block (N.B.)*
1. Median eyebrow san chiku tsuan-tsu	headache eye pain psychosis	Suprorbital and supratrochlear N.B. (Fig. 120)
2. Infraorbital koyroy	trigeminal neuralgia upper toothache	Infrorbital N.B. (Fig. 120)
3. Infratemporal gekan hsia-kuan	trigeminal neuralgia toothache dizzness dislocation of mandible	Maxillary N.B. (2nd branch of trigeminal nerve) Mandibular N.B. (3rd branch of trigeminal nerve) (Fig. 120)
4. High lateral trapezius fuchi fengs-chih	headache tinnitus insomnia occipital pains	Occipital N.B. (Fig. 121)
5. Inframastoid imei I-ming	tonsillitis tinnitus cervical pain	2nd cervical N.B. (Fig. 121)
6. Supraspinatus tenso	shoulder pain breast disease	Suprascapular N.B. (Fig. 121)
7. Axilla kyokusen chi-chuan	shoulder pain intercostal neuralgia neurosis	Brachial plexus N.B. (axillary approach) (Fig. 122)
8. Radial antecubital shiyaku taku ch'in-che	elbow and upper arm pain cough	Radial N.B. (at elbow) (Fig. 122)
9. Ulnar antecubital shyo kai shao-hai	elbow pain neckache, fever toothache, lower leg pain	ulnar N.B. (Fig. 122)
10. Antecubital shyakutaku chih-che	elbow and upper pain cough pharyngitis	Median N.B. (at elbow) (Fig. 123)

Meridian Point *(English)* *(Japanese)* *(Chinese)*	*Effect*	*Nerve Block (N.B.)*
11. Ulnar volar wrist shinmon shen-men	wrist joint pain ulnar nerve pain heart disease insomnia constipation	Ulnar N. B. (at wrist) (Fig. 124)
12. Mid-volar wrist tairyo ta-lin	heart disease dyspnea G.I. pathology wrist joint pain	Median N.B. (at wrist) (Fig. 125)
13. C7-T1 daitsui ta-chui	neck pain asthma psychosis headache malaria	Cervical epidural N.B. (median approach) (Table VI, Fig. 126)
14. T1-T2 todo t'ao-tao	neckache arm and chest muscle disorders headache	Thoracic epidural N.B. (median approach) (Table VI, Fig. 126)
15. L2-L3 meimon ming-men	lumbar disorders impotence G.U. disorders	Lumbar epidural N. B. (Table VI, Fig. 126)
16. Para T3-T4 haiyo fei-yu	pulmonary disorders cough asthma	Thoracic, paravertebral, sympathetic and somatic N.B. (Table VI, Fig. 126)
17. Para T5-T6 (heart) shinyu hsin-yu	cardiac disorder hypertension rheumatism acute psychosis	Thoracic, paravertebral, sympathetic and comatic N.B. (Table VI, Fig. 126)
18. Para T7-T8 (diaphragm) kakuyu ke-yu	esophageal pathology pleuritis epigastric diseases upper G.I. bleeding upper backache	Thoracic, paravertebral, sympathetic and somatic N.B. (Table VI, Fig. 126)
19. Para T9-T10 (liver) kanyu kenye	hepatic disorders intercostal neuralgia insomnia backache	Thoracic, paravertebral, sympathetic and somatic N.B. (Table VI, Fig. 126)

Meridian Point *(English)* *(Japanese)* *(Chinese)*	*Effect*	*Nerve Block (N.B.)*
20. Para T10-T11 (gallbladder) tanyu tan-yu	gallbladder hepatitis backache	Thoracic, paravertebral, sympathetic and somatic N.B. (Table VI, Fig. 126)
21. Para T11-T12 (spleen) hiyu pi-yu	stomach ache anemia indigestion diabetes backache	Thoracic, paravertebral, sympathetic and somatic N.B. (Table VI, Fig. 126)
22. Para T12-L1 (stomach) Iyu wei-yu	G.I. diseases backache	Lumbar, paravertebral, sympathetic and somatic N.B. (Table VI, Fig. 126)
23. Para L2-L3 jinyu shen-yu	renal disorder impotence mental disorders backache	Lumbar, paravertebral, sympathetic and somatic N.B. (Table VI, Fig. 126)
24. Para L3-L4 daichyo yu ta-chang-yu	backache colon disorder skin disorder	Lumbar, paravertebral, sympathetic and somatic N.B. (Table VI, Fig. 126)
25. Lateral L2-L3 shishitsu chih-shih	G.U. disorders reproductive organ disorders	Celiac Plexus N.B. (Table VI)
26. Sacral foramen kyo ryo	sciatic neuralgia backache GYN disorders hemiplegia	Trans-sacral N.B. (Table VI)
27. 2nd Sacral foramen ji ryo tsu-liao	reproductive system disorders backache sciatica	Trans-sacral N.B. (Table VI)
28. Median femoral yin ren yin-lien	reproductive system disorders obturator neuralgia	Obturator N.B. (Fig. 127)

Meridian Point (English) (Japanese) (Chinese)	*Effect*	*Nerve Block (N.B.)*
29. Femoral shyo mon	hip pain reproductive system disorders hernia colic	Femoral N.B. (Fig. 128)
30. Mid gluteal fold shiyofu cheng-fu	sciatica backache hip joint pain	Sciatic N.B. (at gluteal fold) (Fig. 129)
31. Anterior upper fibula yoryosen yang-lin-chuan	leg ache pleuritis paralysis of leg hypertension	Common peroneal N.B. (at neck of bibula) (Fig. 130)
32. Posterior upper tibia inryosen yin-lin-chuan	abdominal distension urinary retention edema and pain of knee leg pain menstrual abnormality	Saphenous N.B. (Fig. 130)
33. Anterior median ankle	leg pain neck pain leg cramp	Deep peroneal N.B. (at angle) (Fig. 130)

34. Scapulocostal Syndrome (Figs. 131, 132):

This is a chronic pain syndrome at the neck, shoulder, back and upper arm. Etiology of this chronic pain is due to posture (Postural Strain). By lowering one shoulder, spinatus scapulae and rheumatoid muscles are pulled constantly. Thus cellulitis and fascitis are developed near the area where the scapula is attached. Tender points are located at the superior median aspect of the scapula and the radiating pain or trigger point is located on the direct of C4, C5, C6, C7, and T1.

Acupuncture points at this area are exactly on the distribution of these nerves where radiating pain is usually existing.

35. "Posterior Mid-Thigh":

Application of an acupuncture needle at the "posterior mid-thigh" point indicates a direct stick of sciatic nerve (Fig. 133).

CHAPTER 5

PROPOSED RESEARCH

OUTLINE OF RECOMMENDATION BY NIH AD HOC COMMITTEE ON ACUPUNCTURE

I. *Surgical Anesthesia* (Dr. Bonica, Chairman—Ad hoc committee—NIH)

A. Clinical Examination.
   1. Neurological and anatomic examination.
   2. Respiratory, hemodynamic and gastrointestinal state.
   3. Metabolic and endocrine state.
   4. Muscle relaxation.
   5. Psychological state.

B. Factors influencing the patient's response.
   1. Relation to hypnotizobility.
   2. Role of training and preconditioning.
   3. Role of relation between patient and physician.
   4. Role of physician and his training.
   5. Role of confusion, understanding and age.
   6. Effect of combined drug therapy and acupuncture.

C. History of Non Chemical Method of Anesthesia.

D. Social and Economical Factor of Acupuncture Anesthesia.

E. Investigations on the Man Under Acupuncture Anesthesia.
   1. Neurological, including Electroencephalogram evoked potential depth recording.
   2. State of hemeostatic mechanism.

F. Study of Animals Under Acupuncture Anesthesia;
   Neurological Study Including Depth Recording and Behavioral Studies.

G. Adequate Chinical Testing.
   1. Exact point of needle insertion, localization and size of effected area.
   2. Influence of the patient's knowledge and belief.
   3. Influence of the physician's knowledge and belief.

4. Role of distant versus close needle insertion with relation to the point of incision.
5. Role of electrical stimulation close or far from the incision points.
6. Independent assessment of results.

II. *Certain Chronic Pain States* (Dr. Bonica, Chairman—Ad hoc committee—NIH)

A. Development of a Therapeutic Trial Procedure.
   1. Patient is trained to describe his pain on scale.
   2. Effect of acupuncture is compared with other therapy.
   3. Therapy is given with suggestion and counter-suggestion.
   4. Questioning of patient is conducted by independent observer.
   5. Time course of the effect is recorded.
   6. Studies at pre and post treatment activities and performance levels.

B. Studies of General State.
   1. Neurological.
   2. Metabolic.
   3. Psychological.

C. Socio-Economic Studies.

D. Studies of Personality and Social Environment of Patients Who Respond to Therapy and Those Who Do Not Or Who Respond Initially But Who Fail to React at Later Stage.

CONSENT FOR MEDICAL PROCEDURES INCLUDING PATHOPHYSIOLOGICAL EVALUATION OF ACUPUNCTURE AND ACUPUNCTURE ANESTHESIA

Hahnemann Hospital Date ____________________

A.M.
Patient ______________ Age ____ Time ____ P.M. Marital Status______

1. I hereby authorize ______________________ and/or Associates and
(Name of Physician)
Assistants to perform upon me medical procedures including pathophysiological evaluation of acupuncture and acupuncture anesthesia.
2. I consent to the performance of operations and procedures in addition to or different from those above which the aboved named doctor and/or associates and assistants may consider necessary or advisable during the course of the above procedure.
3. I understand that the procedure of pathophysiological evaluation of acupuncture and acupuncture anesthesia includes the placing of a very small metalic needle into the specific points of the skin. This is determined by physical examination with or without skin resistance measurement. The points are continuously stimulated by movement

of the needle or application of low voltage electric current needle. Although this procedure has been commonly used in China and Japan, and some of the European Countries, it is entirely experimental here in the United States.

4. I understand that in my consent for pathophysiological evaluation of acupuncture and acupuncture anesthesia the procedure includes the removal of very small metalic needle from the specific points of the skin. For this procedure I grant permission.
5. I understand that the metalic needles are so small a minimum of discomfort can be expected.
6. I understand that this treatment, if successful, may reduce my pain and discomfort, but I am aware and have been advised that neither the hospital nor the physicians can guarantee the success of this treatment.
7. I understand that alternative procedures for the same purpose may be the use of pain killers, intramuscular injections of steroids and/or physical therapy, or surgery.
8. The nature and purpose of the medical procedure including pathophysiological evaluation of acupuncture and acpuncture anesthesia and/or procedures involving alternative methods of diagnosis and treatment, the risk involved, the possibility of complications, and the consequences of the procedure have been fully explained to me. I acknowledge that no guarantee or assurance has been made as to the results that may be obtained. I further acknowledge that I have been informed that because of the experimental nature of the medical procedure, including pathophysiological evaluation of acupuncture and acupuncture anesthesia, of the potential hazards and risks, if any, are not know and cannot be predicted or anticipated by my physician.

____

(Name of Physician)

9. But I nevertheless consent to undergo such potential unknown risks, if any, complications or hazards, if any, to my health. I understand that I may ask any questions concerning the medical procedures including pathophysiological evaluation of acupuncture and acupuncture anesthesia.
10. I understand that I am free at any time to withdraw from or discontinue participation in this study.
11. On my behalf and on behalf of my executor, administrator, and heirs I consent to the taking and publication of any photographs in the course of the operation or procedures for the purpose of advancing medical education. I consent to the examination, photographic studies, and

disposal of any tissues or parts which may be removed by authorities of the Hahnemann Medical College and Hospital.

12. I have been informed that the Hahnemann Medical College and Hospital has filed an assurance with the United States Department of Health, Education, and Welfare and that is available for inspection on request.
13. I have been informed that the United States Department of Health, Education, and Welfare's policy for the protection of human subjects is available for review on request.
14. I certify that I have read and fully understand the above consent statement which has been preceded by an explanation by my physician.

____
(Name of Physician)

that the explanations therein referred to were made to me by

____
(Name of Physician)

and are understood by me, and that all blanks or statements requiring insertion or completion were filled in before I signed.

(CROSS OUT ANY PARAGRAPHS ABOVE WHICH DO NOT APPLY)

Signature ______________________________ Date ____________________
(Patient or Person Authorized to Consent For Patient Stating Relationship of Such Person to Patient)

Signature ______________________________ Date ____________________

Witness ______________________________ Date ____________________

Witness ______________________________ Date ____________________

GENERAL EVALUATION FORM

(Filled Out By Patient And Then Permanent Sheet Typed by Receptionist)

Name	*Age*	*Religion*
Address	*Sex*	*Occupation*
Phone No.	*Race*	*Marital Status*
Referring Physician(s)	*Blue Cross No.*	
Address	*Blue Shield No.*	
Phone No.	*Other Insurance*	
	Medicare No.	
	DPA No.	

Name of Closest Relative	*Employer*
Address	*Address*
Phone No.	*Phone No.*

A. *COMPLETE PAIN HISTORY*
1. Primary Disease Process
2. Onset of Pain and Frequency
3. Nature of Pain and Duration
4. Significant relations to time, position, temperature changes, activities and any unusual parameters elicited from the patient
5. Medications past and present—dosage, frequency, efficacy.
6. Other modes of pain relief—nerve block, steroids, surgery—how effective initially and for how long
7. Degree of incapacity due to pain

B. *SIGNIFICANT PAST MEDICAL HISTORY INCLUDING:*
1. Allergy to drugs
2. Hx of liver disease, especially hepatitis
3. Coagulation disorder
4. Cardiac disease
5. Peripheral vascular disease
6. Diabetes
7. Any neurologic entity giving rise to a sympathetic dyautonomia
8. Alcoholism, any addiction

C. *SIGNIFICANT FAMILY AND SOCIAL HISTORY*
See attached outline of *Social Work in an Acupuncture Study Program*

A. *PHYSICAL EXAM*
Temperature ______ Height ______
Pulse ____________ Weight ______
Blood Pressure __________________

____

I. Skin
II. Heent
III. Cardiac
IV. Pulmonary
V. Abdominal
VI. Neurological
VII. Vascular
VIII. Rectal, Pelvic, Genitalia
IX. Musculo-skeletal

SPECIAL NOTE
1. *Specific Tender Areas:*
2. *Aggravation or Relief by Change of Position:*

1. *Impression of Pain Status:*
2. *Opinion As to Need for Acupuncture:*
3. *Opinion As to Whether Acupuncture will help:*

LABORATORY DATA

Routine (First Visit)
CBC
Differential
Eosinophile count
Austrian Antigen
Urinalysis
EEG—Baseline
SMA—12
Sedimentation Rate
Evoked Potentials
C-reactive Protein

Special
Any indicated X-Rays
EKG if indicated
EMG
Nerve Conduction Time
Electrolytes
Blood Gases
17-OH and KETO Steroids
Plasma Cortisol
Serum Catecholamines
CSF-cell count, Differential
  sugar
  culture
  protein
  catecholamines
CPK
LE Prep
Anti-nuclear Antibody

Follow-up
C-reactive Protein
Eosinophile Count (each visit)
Sedimentation Rate (each visit)
EEG at monthly or bimonthly intervals
Evoked Potential

CONSULTANT'S REPORT

A. *PRE-ACUPUNCTURE*

B. *FOLLOW-UP*

SPECIFIC EVALUATION FORM CHRONIC NECK, SHOULDER, AND ARM PAIN CHRONIC BACK PAIN

DR. J. OSTERHOLM, and DR. G. MATHEWS

At large University centers such as Hahnemann it is quite common to see patients with chronic back pain, neck pain, and headache of cervical origin who have been treated elsewhere with either little or no success. When confronted with these patients many times there is not much to offer them surgically or pharmacologically since they have already been through the whole gamut several times.

A second type of patient is one who has had a recent onset of neck or low back problems to such an extent that they are partially incapacitated and cannot adequately perform at their jobs. Very often their examination and lab studies are minimally abnormal. They are generally treated in a conservative fashion, but they are prone to frequent recurrences of the symptoms.

These are the types of patients we feel might be helped by either Acupuncture alone or in conjunction with other therapeutic modalities.

Therefore, the following protocols have been designed to evaluate these types of patients to be referred for Acupuncture.

NECK, SHOULDER, ARM: EVALUATION SHEET
Patient's Name:
Address:
Telephone No.: Age:

HISTORY
Distribution of neck and shoulder pain:
Distribution of arm-hand symptoms:
Headache: (location, frequency, ocular pain)
Low Back Pain: Leg Pain:
Visual Problems: Dizzy Spells:
Onset of probable cause: (auto-accident, whiplash, diving, fall-off horse, etc.)
Occupation:
Habits: (high pillow, unusual TV watching position)
Duration of Neck Symptoms ____ Arm Symptoms ____ Headache ____
Type of Treatment: Date Location Results

Tests:

Present Medication:
Past Medication:
Level of Function:
Compensation and Insurance Claim Aspects:
Psychiatric History:
Allergic History:
Sphincter and Sex Function:
Examination:
General Status:
Anxiety State:
Stance of Head and Neck:
Muscle Spasm and Tenderness:
Spine Tenderness:
Brachial Plexus Tenderness:
Neck Movements:

Power:	Deltoid	Biceps	Grips	Wrist ext.	Triceps	Hip Flex.
Right						
Left						

Reflexes:	Pectoral	Biceps	Radial	Triceps	KJ	AJ	Plantar	Leg Tone
Right								
Left								

Sensory: (Detailed exam of all major modalities)

BACK PAIN: EVALUATION SHEET
Patient's Name:
Address
Telephone No.: Age:

HISTORY
Diagram of distribution of pain: (Shade darker to indicate more severe pain)
Nature of Pain: (Aching, burning, cutting, etc.)
Duration of Pain:

Type of Treatment:	Date	Location	Results

Tests: (Give approximate dates)
Present Medication:
Past Medication: (Analgesics, Narcotics, Psychotherapeutics)
Occupation: (Past and present)
Present level of function: (Use objective measure, e.g. can walk 3 blocks, etc.)
Compensation or Insurance Claim Aspect:
Psychiatric History:
Sphincter and Sex Functions:

Examination:
General Status:
Anxiety Level:
Stance:
Gait:
Muscle Spasm:
Tenderness: (Spine)

Movement: (Forwards, backwards, rotation, lateral flexion)

	SLR	Lasegues	Hip Extension
Right			
Left			

Power:	Hip Flex	Knee Ext.	Ankle Ext.	Toe Ext.	Ankle Flex	Knee Flex Hip Ext.
Right						
Left						

Reflexes:	KJ	AJ	Hams	Plantars
Right				
Left				

Sensory: (Detailed exam of all major modalities)

RHEUMATOID ARTHRITIS

DR. R. KITRIDOU

Materials and Methods

Patients with classical or definite rheumatoid arthritis and with active synovitis of the finger joints, wrists or knees, will be selected for participation in the study, after signing an appropriate consent form. Pretreatment x-rays will be taken unless these were done within the three months preceding the study. Westergren sedimentation rate and rheumatoid factor (latex fixation)‡ will be performed prior to and at the conclusion of the study.

A. Finger Joints

Actively inflammed joints of one hand will be injected with intraarticular triamcinolone hexacetonide, while the contralateral hand will be treated with acupuncture.

The methods of evaluation of the efficacy of treatment will be the following:

1. Grip strength
2. Tenderness (Dolorimeter score)§—subjective pain (scale 0-3)
3. Ring sizes (PIP and DIPS, 1st MCP)
4. Range of motion (See attached evaluation form)

B. Wrist or Knee Joints

Again one joint will be injected with triamcinolone hexacetonide, while the contralateral will be treated with acupuncture.

Evaluation of treatment efficacy will include:

1. Tenderness (scale 0-3, dolorimeter)—subjective pain (scale 0-3)
2. Heat (scale of 0-3, thermocouple)
3. ROM
4. Circumference

---

*D. J. McCarty: "Treatment of rheumatoid joint inflammation with triamcinolone hexacetonide," *Arthritis Rheum,* 15:157 (1972).

†T. Matsumoto and M. Hayes: "Clinical evaluation of acupuncture for chronic pain. Neuromuscular pain due to degenerative osteoarthritis." Submitted for publication.

‡J. M. Singer and C. M. Plotz: "The latex-fixation test. 1. Application to serologic diagnosis of rheumatoid arthritis," *Am J Med,* 21:888 (1956).

§D. J. McCarty, R. A. Gatter, and P. Phelps: "A dolorimeter for quantification of articular tenderness," *Arthritis Rheum,* 8:551, 1965.

EVALUATION SHEET

FINGER JOINTS

RIGHT LEFT

Grip strength (mm Hg)

Dolorimeter score

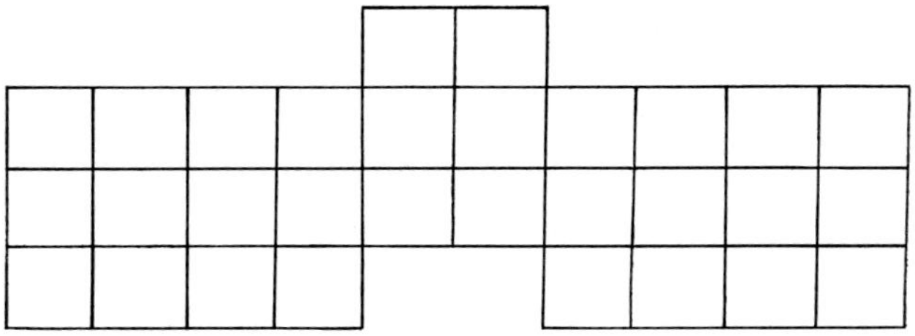

Pain 0 1 2 3 0 1 2 3

Ring sizes

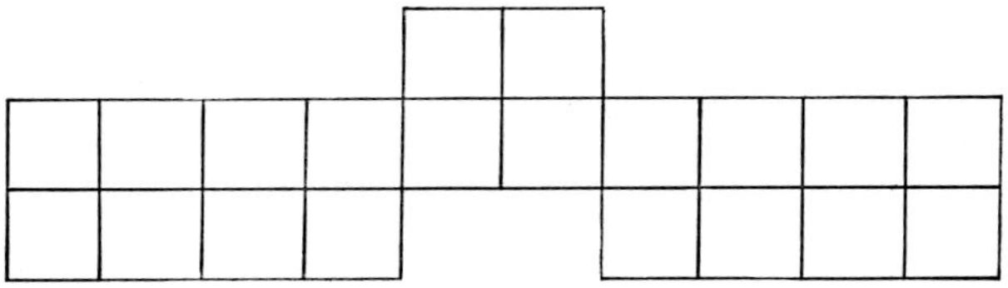

Range of motion

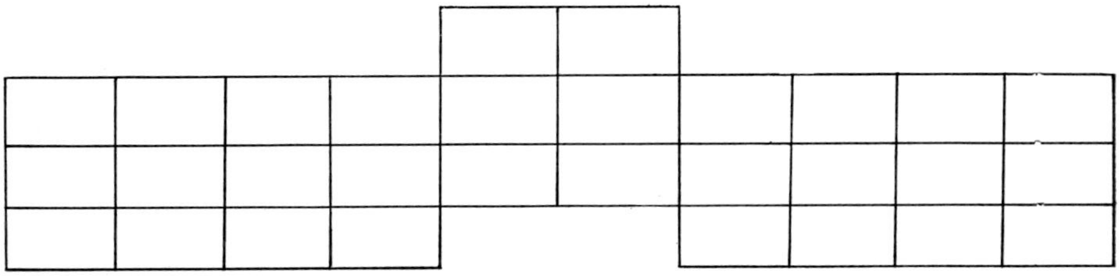

5. Synovianalysis (whenever applicable)
   (See evaluation form)

The above plan of evaluation will permit the detection of any effect of acupuncture on inflammation and synovial thickening, aside from its potential effect on pain.

EVALUATION SHEET

WRISTS KNEES (CIRCLE)

	RIGHT				LEFT			
Tenderness-								
Dolorimeter*								
Observer	0	1	2	3	0	1	2	3
Subjective pain	0	1	2	3	0	1	2	3
Heat								
Thermocouple								
Observer	0	1	2	3	0	1	2	3
Range of motion								
Circumference (cm)								
Synovianalysis								

*Dolorimeter score in the knee joint is derived from measurement on 4 points about the patella, and expressed as the sum of the measurements divided by 4.

The patients will be followed weekly by the Rheumatologist with the determination of the above parameters at each visit, for eight consecutive weeks. The follow-up for the acupuncture will be determined by Dr. Matsumoto.

Evaluation of Results

As long as there is a significant number of patients (and joints), an attempt at statistical evaluation of the results will be made.

THE NEUROPHYSIOLOGICAL ASPECTS OF ACUPUNCTURE STUDY

DR. R. GREEN

The purpose of this section is the study of the neurophysiological and neuroanatomical basis of acupuncture. As acupuncture appears to involve alteration of sensory appreciation (particularly painful sensation) probably through the introduction of additional sensory input and subsequent alteration of afferent impulses from nearby or distant sites consistent with the modern theories of sensory appreciation through peripheral receptors and conductors and essential polysynaptic systems with multiple modulating and influential effects at the synaptic levels of transmission to the somatomotor cortex, it is proposed to study the effect of acupuncture on known physiological sensory potentials of the peripheral and central nervous system.

Since electrical potentials can be evoked by electrical stimulation of pure sensory nerves, such as the sural nerve, or the digital nerves of the extremities (commonly used in clinical neurophysiological practice—digital nerves of the hand), it is proposed that these potentials be studied both in controls and in subjects undergoing acupuncture. It is further proposed that these evoked sensory potentials also be studied in animal subjects, again utilizing controls and acupuncture-treated animals.

The amplitude of these evoked pure sensory potentials is extremely small, seldom exceeding 50 uV at the distal site and becoming smaller as the potential reaches the more proximal peripheral nervous system structures and as the impulse passes through the polysynaptic ascending pathways to the somatosensory cortex. Consequently, it is necessary to use extremely sensitive amplifying equipment and analog to digital computation methods in order to accurately and precisely analyze these potentials at the appropriate locations. Precise time-locked stimulators are also necessary to produce accurate stimulating potentials, and high quality tape recording systems are required for storage and review of collective data.

More specifically, it is proposed that sensory potentials be produced by stimulation of the digital nerves of the fingers utilizing ring electrodes with analysis of the evoked potential at the wrist, at a more proximal site (probably the elbow), and at a further proximal site (probably over the area of the dorsal root ganglia). It is then proposed to analyze the ascending potential over the spinal cord by the method utilized by Cracco *et al.* and ultimately the somatosensory evoked cortical potential as described in literature by numerous investigations.

It is expected that the evoked potentials will be evaluated in terms of the morphology of the potential, the latency and conduction times of the potentials, possible alterations in the amplitude of the potentials and of their duration. It is further planned to study the influence of other sensory phenomena on the somatosensory evoked potential, again in controls and in subjects undergoing acupuncture anesthesia. The latter include visual, auditory, and probably motor stimulation. It is further proposed to study effects of acupuncture anesthesia upon other sensory evoked potentials such as the auditory and visual evoked potential.

In order to study the neurophysiological and neuroanatomical substrates of acupuncture and algesia it is proposed to perform the following neurophysiological studies in both animals and humans, using the same individuals and control prior to the performance of acupuncture and follow-up *control* in a period following acupuncture if possible. As there is variation from individual to individual in both peripheral and central evoked neurophysiological potentials, there is no advantage to using a separate control group.

The technique for study is essentially identical for both animal and human subjects. In both situations, electrical stimulation will be applied over a peripheral nerve, specifically the median nerve in the right extremity, using stimulating electrodes on the digits in humans and just proximal to the wrist in both humans and animals. In humans sensory evoked potentials will be studied at the wrist and antecubital fossa and only at the antecubital fossa in animals. These potentials will be collected and stored in a Nicolet 1072 analog-digital converter with monitoring both oscilloscopically and by paper write-out. The collected data will then be averaged to produce an averaged evoked potential at the sites described. Similar collection of data will be performed at the more proximal portions of the peripheral nerve at the junction of the dorsal roots with the spinal cord, over the spinal cord ipsilaterally and contralaterally, and over the scalp bilaterally with particular reference to the contralateral somatosensory areas of the brain. The collected averaged potentials will then be written out on an X-Y plotter for visual analysis. Data will also be collected and stored in a high quality multichannel tape recorder for further analysis and exchange of information.

This procedure will be performed prior to acupuncture in all subjects, both animal and human, and then repeated while the subjects are undergoing acupuncture analgesia performed locally in the area of nerve stimulation. The technique will then be repeated with analgesia performed in more remote areas to study the less direct effect of acupuncture analgesia on the sensory and somatomotor evoked potentials.

The level of consciousness of all subjects will be monitored constantly through 8-channel EEG monitor and physiologic parameters such as movement, heart rate and respiration will be constantly monitored.

PSYCHIATRIC PROTOCOL

DR. R. NATHAN

At the initial stage of the investigation, the psychiatrist will perform two separate functions: he will do a psychiatric examination on each patient who, in the clinical judgement of the research team, shows evidence of significant psychiatric disturbance. This group of patients will be interviewed with heavy emphasis being placed on the mental status examination in order to accurately judge the current psychopathological state of the patient. The mental status examination will be recorded with verbatim samples of the patient's speech and thought content included. Especially noted will be the patient's interview behavior including his ability to relate as well as his verbal and non verbal behavior. His affective state will similarly be recorded as well as his content of thought whether there is evidence of abnormal mental trends or hallucinations.

In addition to this, his orientation will be tested as to time, place and person, and recent and remote memory determined. The patient's judgement and reliability will also be determined. Where necessary, family, social and developmental history will be obtained in order to establish a diagnosis. The relationship of the patient's physical complaint to his emotional state will similarly be elicited if it is at all possible.

The second group of patients to be examined will be those who are to be tested in the analgesia section of the study. A number of these patients will be selected at random and referred to me for examination of the dynamic role that chronic pain plays in their life. Where necessary, a differential diagnosis will be attempted between chronic pain of an organic versus chronic pain as a neurotic symptom. In those patients with organic chronic pain, there will be an attempt to clarify the role of the pain in the psychological life of the patient. In particular, we will be looking for those persons to whom the pain represents a necessary aspect of their functional operations, for example those patients to whom the pain represents a needed punishment; those patients to whom pain represents a method by which relationships can be maintained; those persons for whom pain protects them from having to make unpleasant decisions or take feared actions; essentially, then, to try to determine whether the pain represents something from which the patient can obtain secondary gratification. We will try to determine if the individual is using the pain to solve overwhelming current conflicts and in what way the pain has become fused with emotionally charged life situations. Without communicating the findings to the other investigators, records of the dynamic formulations will be kept and when the particular patients have received the treatment and the efficacy of it determined, the psychiatric protocols will be discussed.

After the preliminary phase of the investigation is over, more sophisticated techniques concerning the placebo effect and determination of secondary gain will be instituted with the help of Dr. Orne and Dr. Evans of the University of Pennsylvania, who we have already seen as consultants and who have agreed to become co-investigators.

CLINICAL EVALUATION OF ACUPUNCTURE ANESTHESIA

DR. H. PRICE AND DR. J. PURNELL

Since the first hand reports from China by Doctors Diamond and White, acupuncture as a means of providing surgical anesthesia has become a number one topic both in the lay and anesthesia press. It is difficult for the western oriented physician to accept this new mode of anesthesia which was introduced only a few years ago by the Chinese. If acupuncture does indeed block the normal reactions to surgical pain, it becomes obvious that this entire problem should be thoroughly investigated by qualified and interested personnel.

It is the purpose of the Department of Anesthesiology at Hahnemann Medical College and Hospital to study and explore acupuncture anesthesia as part of a combined effort with the Division of Surgical Research and other Hahnemann Departments to further deliniate and define the place of acupuncture in the practice of medicine.

"This is not Humbug—or is it?" was the editorial view by Nicholas Green in a recent publication of ANESTHESIOLOGY which suggested we keep an "open mind" and "search for data on what might just prove to be a potentially valuable contribution to the field of anesthesiology."

The approach to this problem will be in two forms. First we will work closely with the Pain Clinic in its use of acupuncture in the relief of pain, comparing this method with our more traditional approach of nerve blocks with local anesthesia. Having mastered the technique of acupuncture and its place in the relief of pain, we will then apply this knowledge to the application of acupuncture anesthesia in the operative theatre.

The first series to be studied according to the classification of the American Society of Anesthesiology will be Class 1 and 11 patients with benign skin lesions such as moles, warts, and nevi as well as superficial lipomas and fibromas. Fifteen such patients will be studied in the following manner:

1. Physical examination and history as required by all operative patients.
2. Laboratory tests consisting of blood count, hematocrit, urine analysis, EEG, SMA-12 and other pertinent studies.
3. Complete explanation to the patient of exactly what we plan to do, and signing of the patient consent form.
4. Standby anesthesia—local or general—to be employed if needed. This

is especially important since the good of the patient is our primary concern at all times.

5. No preoperative medication.
6. A postoperative question form to be filled out by all patients regarding their experiences and sensations with acupuncture anesthesia.
7. Postoperative care will be the usual care given to such patients.

The patients will be divided into three groups A, B, and C for surgery and acupuncture anesthesia study.

Group A

Five patients will be studied in the following manner:

1. BP will be recorded with a syphygmomanometer.
2. ECG recorded on a 4 channel monitor and permanently recorded with a *Simultrace* recorder.
3. Analgesia will be determined by the loss of sensation to painful needle stimuli. The area of analgesia will be determined at 10 minute intervals following the onset of acupuncture and will continue for one hour with the areas being mapped out on each patient.
4. The method of acupuncture will be that of manual stimulation.

Group B

Five patients will be studied similar to Group A with the following exceptions:

1. BP will be recorded with an eighteen plastic needle inserted into the radial artery the evening before surgery and displayed on a 4 channel monitor with a permanent record being made with the *Simultrace* recorder.
2. EEG will be recorded.
3. Blood gases pre-operatively, intro-operatively and post-operatively.
4. SMA-12 tests will be drawn before surgery, during surgery and after surgery.
5. Catecholamines studies before and after surgery will be performed as soon as the technique is standardized.
6. Continuous rectal temperature.
7. Acupuncture stimulation will be performed with an American made stimulator.

Group C

Five patients will be studied exactly as Group B except for the method of acupuncture stimulation which will be performed with a Chinese made stimulator.

The following monitoring equipment is available in the operative suite:

1. Seven 4 channel Electronics for Medicine, three trace monitors.
2. Two E for M Simultrace recorders.
3. Six Microdot and six Statham transducers.
4. Two E for M ECG monitors.
5. One 4 channel Hewlitt Packard monitor.
6. One Electrodyne cardiac monitor with cardiac pacemaker and internal-external defibrillator.
7. Two neuromuscular blockade monitors.
8. One blood gas analyzer.
9. CO_2 analyzer (Godart).
10. Grass 8 channel polygraph recorder.
11. Nine temperature probes and recorders.

SOCIAL SERVICE ACTIVITIES

MR. J. SIMMONS

The purpose of this study has been stated to be "to evaluate the feasibility of acupuncture—to develop an acceptable standard technique—and to evaluate side effects and complications." Social Work will become involved in several areas of this study on a professional level (the Social Worker will have a Master's Degree in Social Work). These areas are: (1) Direct Counseling Service, (2) Referral and (3) Research.

Direct Counseling Service

Because of the widespread interest in the use of acupuncture large numbers of people are flocking to existing services for a *cure*. Careful screening of patients is planned so that those people who are emotionally stable and realistically oriented to the possibilities of acupuncture can be placed in the program. The Graduate Social Worker will interview each applicant and assist the other team members in evaluating potential members. Careful attention will be paid to past medical treatment attempts (as for example, the patient gone from doctor to doctor looking for the impossible cure), the patient's feelings about his medical problems and his feelings regarding the use of acupuncture.

After the patient has been accepted into the program supportive counseling will continue around the patient's feelings regarding his progress (or lack of it) and in general the adjustments the patient will be making in terms of his personal life throughout treatment. Family members will be involved in this process as well since the families interaction can aid or impede the progress of medical treatment.

Throughout the course of treatment information regarding all of the above will be shared with the team as it relates to the patient's medical progress so that maximum potentials can be achieved.

If the individual is not accepted into the Acupuncture Program other referrals will be made. These might include the resources mentioned above, Community Mental Health Services and other clinics that would be more appropriate to the patient's needs.

Referrals

Whether or not a patient is not accepted to the program appropriate referrals will be made. During treatment referrals for financial assistance, boarding homes, vocational rehabilitation, and other community agencies might need to be made. The Graduate Social Worker will be responsible for this component.

Research

Several areas of social data will be quite important as the study hopes to develop a wealth of information in the area of acceptance of acupuncture by the patient. Will it effect all people the same or is there a typical type of individual for whom acupuncture will or will not work? For example, will a highly educationed person not respond to treatment? As a part of the Social Work interviewing process, questions regarding the patient's economic, educational, occupational, religious and social class background will be explored in an attempt to determine average profiles if any do exist.

In summary, the Graduate Social Worker (MSW) will be of service in the screening process, in counseling as the program progresses, in referral to other needed kinds of service and in establishing social profiles. The Graduate Social Worker is a vital member of the team.

A PATHOPHYSIOLOGIC MODEL OF ACUPUNCTURE WITH RESPECT TO PAIN RELIEF AND ANESTHESIA

DR. V. AMBRUSO

Background

Initially the concept of pain perception was attributed to stimulation of specific receptors and free nerve endings in the skin and deeper levels, and transmitted to the thalamus and cortex via the spinothalamic tracts. With the advent of surgical procedures for pain it became obvious that other pathways were involved. These were at the cord level in a paramedial ascending system of the reticular system which projected to the medially placed nuclei of the Thalamus. Also, subcortical structures, principally the Limbic system, were also shown to have varied effects on pain syndromes.

In 1965 Melzack and Wall published their now famous work on the Gate Control Theory of Pain. (Fig. 134)

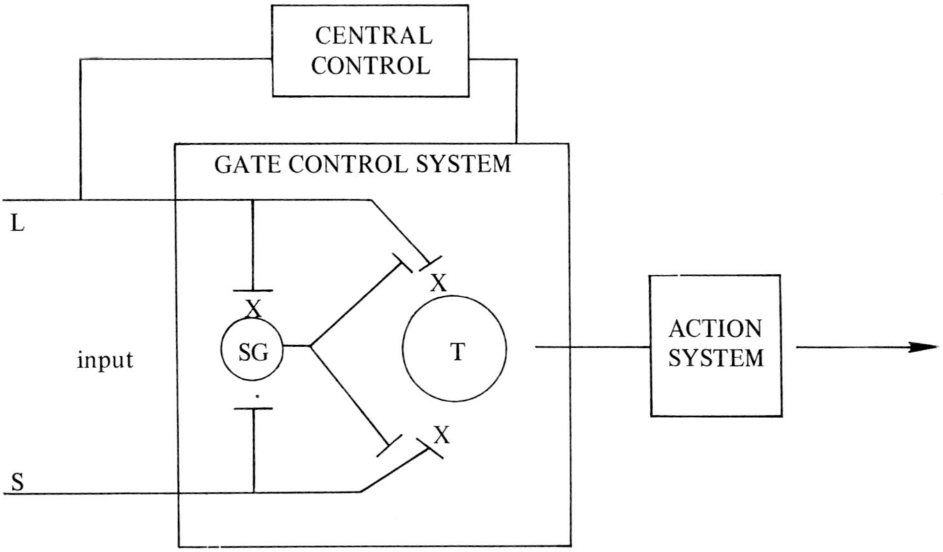

Figure 134: Schema for gate control theory of pain

In Sweet and White's latest edition of *PAIN AND THE NEUROSURGEON,* Dr. Sweet and Dr. White describe a series of patients with varied pain lesions (Peripheral Neuralgias, Trigeminal Neuralgia, Atypical Facial Neuralgia, and Oropharyngeal pain). All of these but the last were treated with electrical stimulation of the involved nerves with generally good results. They attribute their success to stimulation of the large fibers. These fibers in turn stimulated the cells in the substantia gelatinosa which in turn inhibited the smaller fibers carrying the painful stimuli to the transmitter cell.

This small series of cases has encouraged us to undertake further investigation along these lines, since we feel that acupuncture is a form of stimulation acting on the larger fibers producing inhibition at the level of the Gate.

Experimental Methods and Data

Medium size albino rabbits were restrained in a supine position and both manual and electrical stimuli were applied at various points. Acupuncture needles were placed percutaneously in all of the web spaces of fore and hind paws individually and stimulated. A second needle was always placed at the vertex. The most successful model which produced consistent anesthesia of the thorax, abdomen, and upper portions of all four extremities was with:

i. manual-simultaneous stimulation of a needle in the index web and vertex.

ii. electrical-a sine wave current at 10,000 cps with 200 microamperes was conducted via a needle in the index web to a needle at the vertex.

The electrical stimulation was superior to the manual. Also, when the direction of the current was reversed, and sent from vertex to index web the result was quite poor.

We now propose to do discrete dissection of the nerve fibers in the index and other webs as well as larger peripheral nerves, and stimulate them directly as described previously.

Preliminary Conclusions

We feel that our data strengthens the concept of the Gate Theory, especially in reference to our electrical stimulation experiments. In these the direction of the current was a critical factor. It essentially was conducted from the periphery toward the cord and higher centers, and we feel directly affected the gate located in the substantia gelantinosa.

Goals

Hopefully we will be able to show that our concept on the Pathophysiologic Mechanism of Acupuncture is correct. To substantiate this concept we plan to undertake sophisticated neurophysiologic monitoring, especially EEG and sensory evoked potentials in both animals and humans. Our studies will include both Acupunctures Analgesia and Anesthesia. All of the monitoring will be done on normal controls and pathologic models before, during, and after acupuncture. Each group will be studied using both manual and electrical methods of stimulation. In addition the electrical portion of the study will be carried out in a double blind manner so that the data obtained can be evaluated more objectively.

Chapter 6

Additional Studies

SECTION 1: PATHOPHYSIOLOGY OF ACUPUNCTURE: NERVOUS SYSTEM TRANSMISSION

(In Collaboration With Bruce Levy, M.D.)

DURING THE PAST 18 MONTHS we have been actively engaged in clinical as well as experimental basic science research. First, regarding the existance of reproducible acupuncture analgesia which we have been able to establish, and second, the pathophysiology of its analgesic properties.

Over one year ago we had no idea how to produce acupuncture analgesia in the research laboratories.[89] Through a slow trial and error, procedure, we determined that the more peripherally placed the needle, on the animal, the greater the degree of analgesic could be obtained. However, this was not the only factor because a needle placed and manually stimulated in the second web space of the paw would produce a great deal of analgesia while that in the third paw web space would produce much less analgesia.

We then selectively, manually stimulated the different anatomic structures in these areas, and found that almost no analgesia could be obtained by stimulating bone, muscle or tendon. However, direct stimulation of the superficial distal radial nerve reproduced the analgesic pattern obtained by cutaneous manual stimulation of the second web of the paw. At this point we had no mechanical device to stimulate the nerves in a reproducible manner.

We acquired an EXACT signal generator which had a means of altering its frequency and its wave form. Again, through trial and error we found the best location to produce analgesia was to have the negative lead on the vertex and the positive lead on the nerve directly. The generator could emit a square, delta and sine wave. All wave forms produced some degree of analgesia but the sine wave set at 10 kilohertz frequency and a current of 200 u amperes produced the best analgesic distribution. After establishing the fact that analgesia could be conclusively reproduced, we then entered the second phase of our research.

By surgically isolating nerves and then applying acupuncture to them we were able to establish a somatic distribution of analgesic pattern which could be established by either manual stimulation or by the People's Republic of China Acupuncture/Anesthesia apparatus 71-1. The area of analgesia was always greater with the machine than by manual stimulation. However, these effects are not solely due to electrical stimulation because manual stimulation always achieved a reproducible analgesic area.

We, thus, decided to work on one single nerve and the sciatic nerve was chosen strictly because of its size and easy accesibility. The following study was established for the purpose of helping to determine the pathophysiology of acupuncture.

Material and Method:

Forty rabbits were divided into ten equal groups of four rabbits each. The facts about each animal grouping are shown in Table VII.

Animals were anesthetized with Diethyl ether by open drop method and the sciatic nerve was exposed. The effects of the anesthetic were allowed to dissipate before any study was then attempted. The animals served as their own controls in that they were tested for pain response before any acupuncture therapy was given.

The People's Republic of China Acupuncture/Anesthesia apparatus 71-1 which emits a pulse in the form of a differentiated type of square wave was used. This apparatus consists of four channels each of which contains two electrode leads, one lead being positively triggered and the other electrode lead triggered negatively (Figure 77). Figure 135 shows the positive trig-

TABLE VII

SCIATIC NERVE PILOT STUDY

Animal Group	*Location of Positive Triggered Electrode*	*Location of Negative Triggered Electrode*	*Disruptive Action on Sciatic Nerve*
1.	Main trunk sciatic nerve	Vertex	None
2.	Vertex	Main trunk sciatic nerve	None
3.	Common tibial nerve	Vertex	None
4.	Vertex	Common tibial nerve	None
5.	Lower portion sciatic nerve trunk	Upper portion sciatic nerve trunk	None
6.	Upper portion sciatic nerve trunk	Lower portion sciatic nerve trunk	None
7.	Sciatic nerve distal portion	Vertex	Nerve severed
8.	Vertex	Sciatic nerve distal portion	Nerve severed
9.	Sciatic nerve main trunk	Vertex	1% procaine directly applied to block the nerve
10.	Vertex	Sciatic Nerve Main	1% procaine directly applied to block the nerve

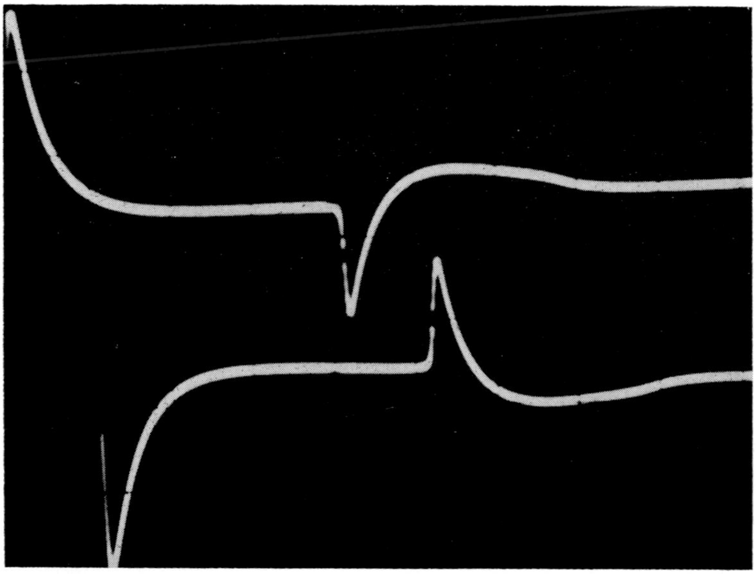

Figure 135: Top: Positive triggered electrode Bottom: Negative triggered electrode (Both from Chinese Acupuncture Apparatus 71-1).

gered pulse as the upper wave form and the negative triggered pulse as the lower wave form.

The positive and negative electrodes were placed on the nerve directly and on the vertex. The animals were tested for pain by first applying

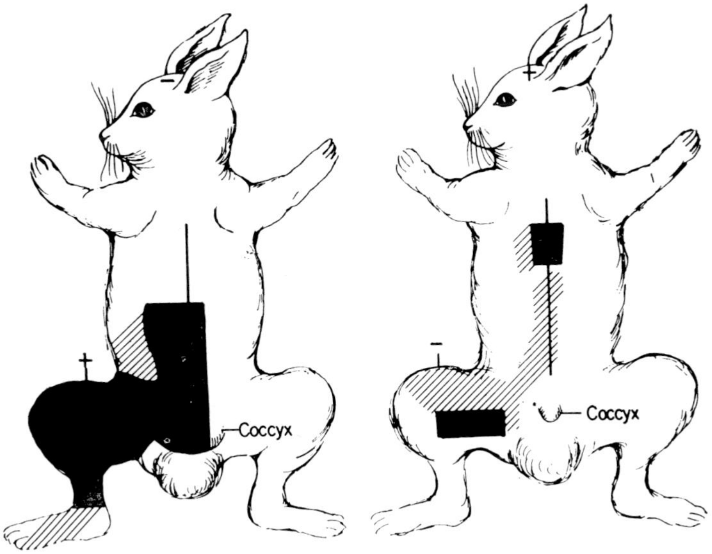

Figure 136: Analgesic patterns obtained with electrodes on the 1 sciatic nerve main trunk and on the vertex.

warm water in the test tube against the skin. If no pain response occurred, then a pinprick with twenty-five gauge needle was used to determine analgesia. If again no pain response was illicited, then a Kocher clamp was applied to these anesthetic areas to insure the validity of analgesis. Once an area showed response to pain, no further painful stimuli were applied to this area. If pain was evoked then a characteristic spike appeared on the electroencephalogram (Figure 89) and the animal showed signs of reflex withdrawal. Electroencephalographic tracings were taken for each animal throughout the procedure.

The animals were retested for pain response to insure that no residual analgesia persisted. Then, the animal was given a second treatment but this time the positive and negative electrodes were switched to discount any residual effects and analgesic areas again were tested. The skin incision on the animal was then sterilely closed, and the animals are being followed for any long term detrimental effects.

Results:

The areas of analgesia obtained are shown in drawing form in Figures 136 through 140. Certain patterns can be ascertained from these figures.

When the positive needle electrode was placed on the peripheral nerve and the negative needle electrode on the vertex, an area of analgesia was obtained which extended beyond the limits of this nerve's anatomical distribution. Analgesia crossed the midline and was recorded into the thoracic

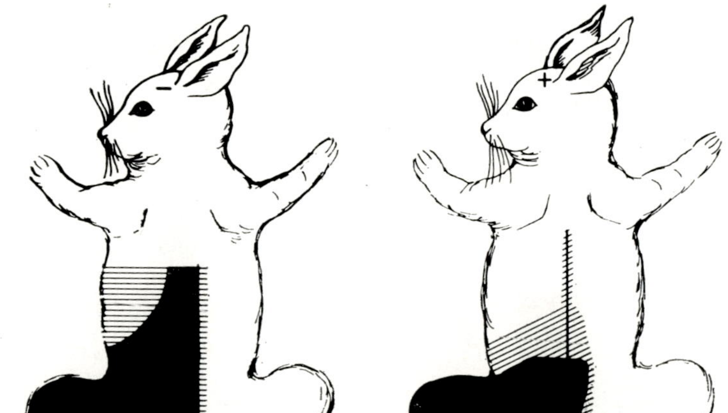

Figure 137: Analgesic patterns obtained with electrodes on the common tibial nerve and on the vertex.

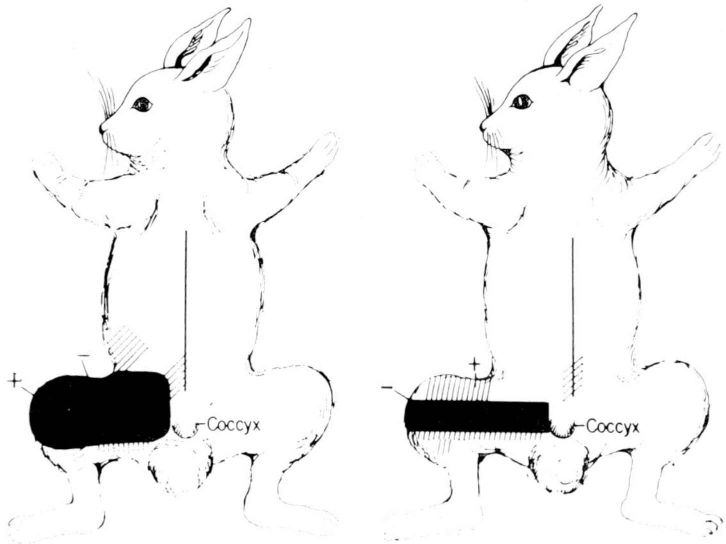

Figure 138: Analgesic patterns obtained with both electrodes on the sciatic nerve separated by a 5 cm distance.

dermatome region as well as in the normal sciatic nerve distribution. When the electrodes were reversed analgesia occurred but to a less extent and in a smaller somatic area as can be seen in Figure 136.

When the positive electrode was placed in the common tibial nerve and

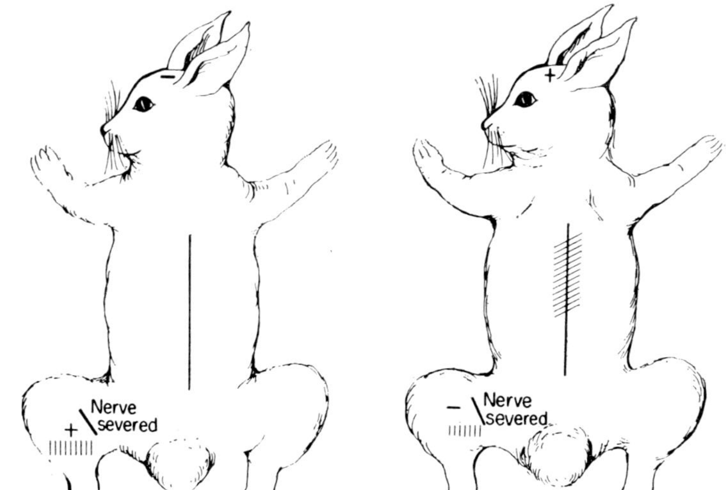

Figure 139: Analgesic pattern obtained with the electrodes on the distal portion of the severed sciatic nerve and the vertex.

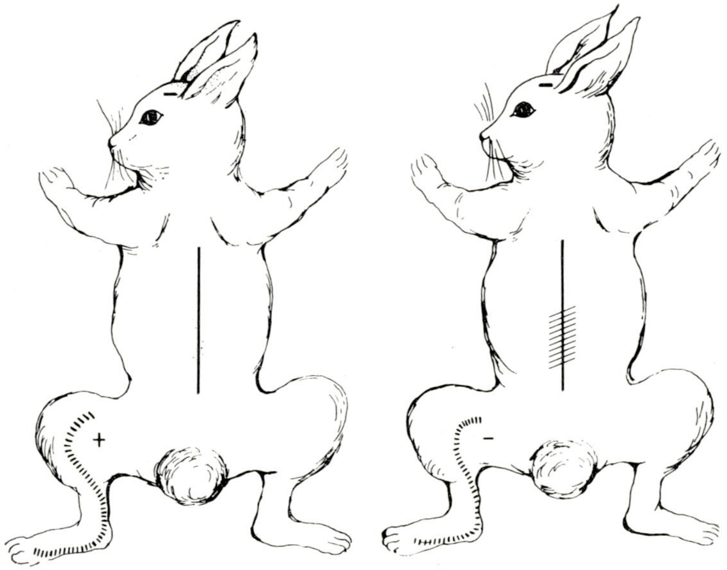

Figure 140: Analgesic pattern obtained with the electrodes on the sciatic nerve main trunk and on the vertex, but first the sciatic nerve was blocked with 1% procaine directly.

the negative electrode in the vertex, the areas of analgesia obtained were greater than those obtained with the sciatic nerve. Analgesia included anatomical nerve distribution, midline overlap, the coccyx, and also extended into the thoracic dermatomes. When the tibial nerve held the negative electrode, analgesia was mostly obtained only in its anatomical distribution.

When both electrodes were placed in the sciatic nerve, only a local area of analgesia occurred corresponding to this nerve's distribution. No analgesia could be obtained when the nerve was precut and the distal portion stimulated. Also analgesia could not be obtained with an intact sciatic nerve when first anesthetized with 1% procaine locally on the nerve and then given an acupuncture treatment.

In addition, the following incidental observations were made. These being that when adequate acupuncture analgesia was obtained there was: first, an increased incidence of bowel movements associated with visible peristaltic waves and high pitched peristaltic sounds; second, that in areas of analgesia there appeared grossly at least to be no evidence of neuromuscular blockade; thirdly, in over 60% of the animals (60 rabbits) a change from a quick beta to a slower beta rhythm occurred and in over 50% of these animals the electroencephalographic pattern converted to an alpha rhythm (Figure 141). No subject began with a normal alpha rhythm or was there any replacement of alpha rhythm by low amplitude fast waves or superimposed upon this rhythm any sleep spindles which would indicate a de-

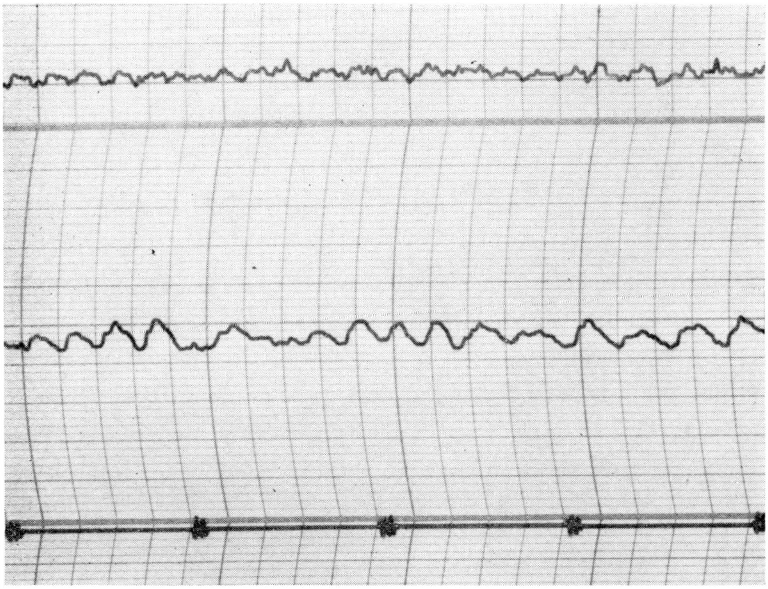

Figure 141: EEG conversion from beta or alpha rhythm: Beta rhythm above; alpha rhythm below after one half hour of acupuncture therapy.

Note: Figures 136 through 140 show cutaneous analgesia obtained upon rabbits after acupuncture treatment. Heavy shading shows total analgesia, stripe show heavy analgesia. All other areas no analgesia. Plus sign refers to the positive triggered electrode needle placement and minus sign refers to the negative triggered electrode needle placement.

crease level of consciousness.[90] Lastly, by varying the placement of the needle along the course of the peripheral nerve, distally and proximally, a greater or lesser degree of analgesic area could be obtained.

Comments:

Certain assumptions can be made from this preliminary study. First, acupuncture is mediated through the nervous system. Secondly, it takes an intact, functioning nervous system for this therapy to be successful. Thirdly, the more distal the nerve is stimulated, the greater degree of analgesia obtained. Fourth, acupuncture analgesia conforms to the distribution of the nerve treated, but it also extends to overlapping areas. Lastly, it requires some contact with the central nervous system for acupuncture analgesia to be maximally successful.

Recent studies from China, reported by H. Jack Geiger, M.D. performed over the last five years indicate some exciting new insights into the theory of how acupuncture works.[91] A number of reputable investigators doing human as well as animal research have found that: first, acupuncture is not due to any form of hypnosis; secondly, although there is no alteration in consciousness and no evidence of cortical depression, acupuncture changes the patient's perception of both the intensity and quality of pain. This is presumably accomplished by specific blocking actions at two and perhaps three levels of the central nervous system. Thirdly, that these blocking actions most likely occur in the internuncial neurons of the posterior horn of the spinal cord and within two distinct thalamic nuclei. A fourth conclusion which they have reached is that acupuncture is mediated through the proprioceptive pathways of the central nervous system.

They reached this conclusion for two reasons. First, after proper acupuncture therapy a phenomenon called Te-chi's occurs. This is a soreness, pain, numbness, heaviness and tingling spreading from the site of acupuncture needling when its analgesic effect begins. We have also observed this phenomenon in our clinical practice and have termed it simply "needle shock" or "needle sensation." Second, novocaine injection into the deep nerve supply of the muscle could block the effect of acupuncture (i.e. raise the pain threshold) but cutaneous novocaine at the site of acupuncture therapy could not block its effects.

We as well as the Chinese researchers believe that acupuncture is not a form of hypnosis, and that it does alter the patient's perception of both the intensity and quality of pain. Although the Chinese explanation for this phenomenon is that specific blocking actions occur at areas in the central nervous system, we hypothesize, that in addition, this aspect of therapy may also partially be the result of a slowing in the electroencephalographic pattern from a beta to alpha rhythm.

It is possible that the blocking action does presumably occur in the central nervous system, especially in the internuncial pool and at the thalamic level. However, this is not a new concept, Drs. Wall and Melzack[4] hypothesized the existence of a minimum of two central nervous system gates in their article on pain mechanisms.

The Chinese believe that acupuncture is propagated through the proprioceptive portion of the nervous system. Their reasons for this conclusion, as stated previously, are because of the Te-chi phenomenon and because of their cutaneous local blockade. This explanation is not tenable to these investigators. Because of our clinical impression of the sensation which the patient describes to us from "Needle Shock" and because of the animal's ability to retain his proprioceptive function after acupuncture anesthesia, we believe that transmission is through the classic pain fiber system of the central nervous system. It is possible that gates exist in the spinal dorsal root ganglion and internuncial neurons which block selectively the impulses going to the spinothalamic tract. Also a second gate or gates exist in the thalamus which allows selective passage of all impulses, but blocks those remaining spinothalamic impulses which have passed through the first gate.

Acupuncture is not a form of suggestion or hypnosis, but it does decrease the patient's conscious perception of pain through this second selective gate located in the thalamus. The other impulses are then normally relayed from the thalamus to the vertex. Pain transmission is blocked by acupuncture and this is the hypothesized reason for analgesia, but proprioceptive transmission persists for transmission of other impulses as shown in the Chinese work.

We are also presently beginning studies on the effects of acupuncture on the autonomic nervous system because of our findings of alterations in gastro-intestinal motality with acupuncture treatment. Another project in which we are now engaged is the study of the ability of acupuncture, in areas of proven analgesia, to have any effect on neuromuscular transmission and to determine if any extent of neuromuscular blockade exists.

Summary:

As far as we know, this is the first scientific report which shows distinctly that acupuncture is transmitted directly by the nervous system and the performance of analgesic acupuncture requires an intact nervous system. The more distal the acupuncture treatment is given upon the nerve, the greater the degree of analgesia is afforded. The slowing from a normal awake beta to a normal awake alpha electroencephlographic rhythm may have some effect on the patient's pain perception but further investigation is required.

SECTION 2: INTESTINAL MOTILITY AND ACUPUNCTURE

(In Collaboration With Victor Ambruso, M.D.)

During The Course Of Our Laboratory investigations into acupuncture anesthesia, we have noticed with considerable frequency the very prominent peristaltic waves moving across the abdominal wall followed by defecation. Associated with this phenomenon were high pitched peristaltic sounds. These observations led to the following investigation of the effect of acupuncture on intestinal motility.

Material and Method:

Twelve albino rabbits five to seven pounds in weight were anesthetized with intravenous pentobarbital in a dosage of 5 mg per pound, and a laparotomy was performed. The stomach was then identified, and through a small incision a small balloon catheter was passed beyond the pylorus and advanced into the proximal jejunum. The catheter was secured to the stomach incision with a purse string suture, and the abdominal cavity closed.

The balloon catheter was then calibrated against a water manometer on a zero to thirty centimeter water pressure scale. The catheter was then connected to the Sanborn recorder via a calibrated pressure transducer for continuous monitoring at a paper speed of 2.5 millimeters per minute. The transducer was calibrated so that each vertical millimeter division on the paper, represented one centimeter of water pressure. Each animal served as its own control with a baseline motility being recorded before any acupuncture or chemical stimuli were applied. The animals were divided into four equal groups of three rabbits each. The first at a constant current of 200 microamperes and at a frequency of 10 kilohertz per second for thirty minutes. All of these nine animals had the negative electrode placed in the right groin via a 21 gauge needle. The acupuncture needles always were attached to the positive electrode. In all nine animals the acupuncture needles were placed in the following eight positions consecutively: 1) right ear; 2) left ear; 3) right index web; 4) left index web; 5) right thumb and 6) left thumb web; 7) right thigh and 8) left thigh. The stimulus was applied only to one point at a time. Then the results were recorded and the curve was allowed to return to its baseline for thirty minutes. Each point was then stimulated in the above order and thirty minute intervals were allowed between each stimulus in order to insure the return of the curve to its baseline. The only difference in the type of stimulus

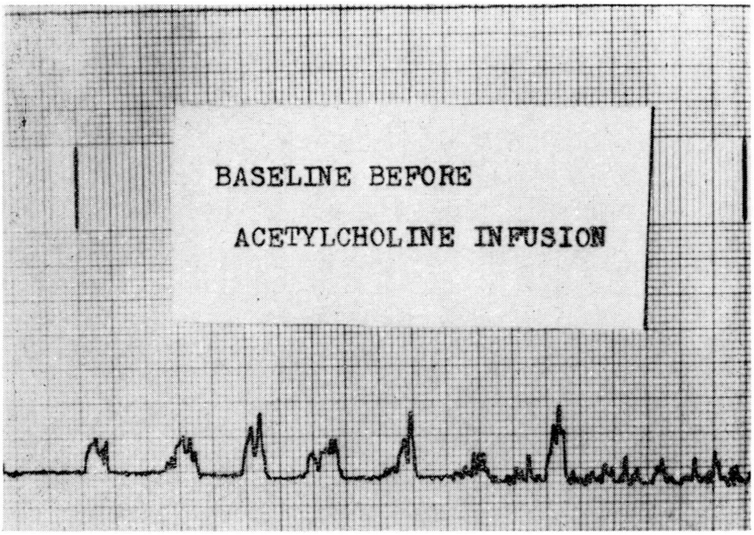

Figure 142: Intestinal motility tracing before acetylcholine infusion.

for these first three groups was the wave form which was delivered by the positive electrode. The first group received a sine wave pulse. The second group received a delta wave pulse and the third group received their stimulus by a square wave pulse. The fourth group of three rabbits did not receive acupuncture, but were given an intravenous infusion of acetylcholine in a dose of 200 ug/kg/mm over thirty minutes.[92]

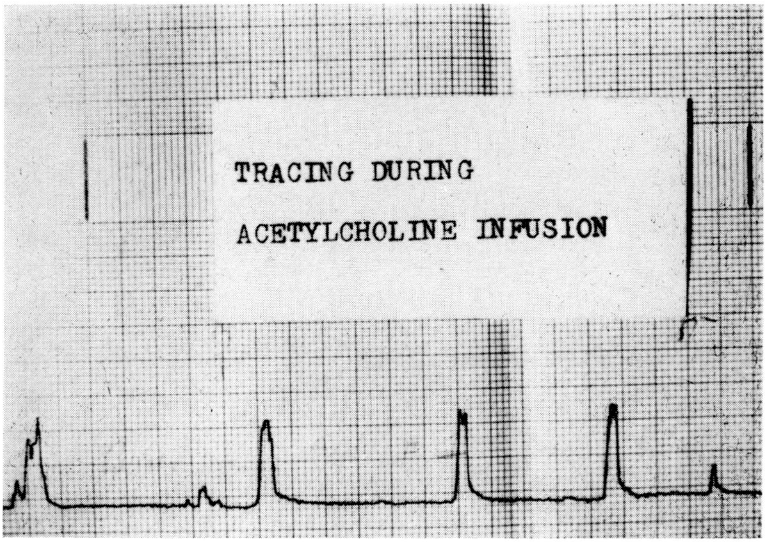

Figure 143: Intestinal motility tracing after acetylcholine infusion.

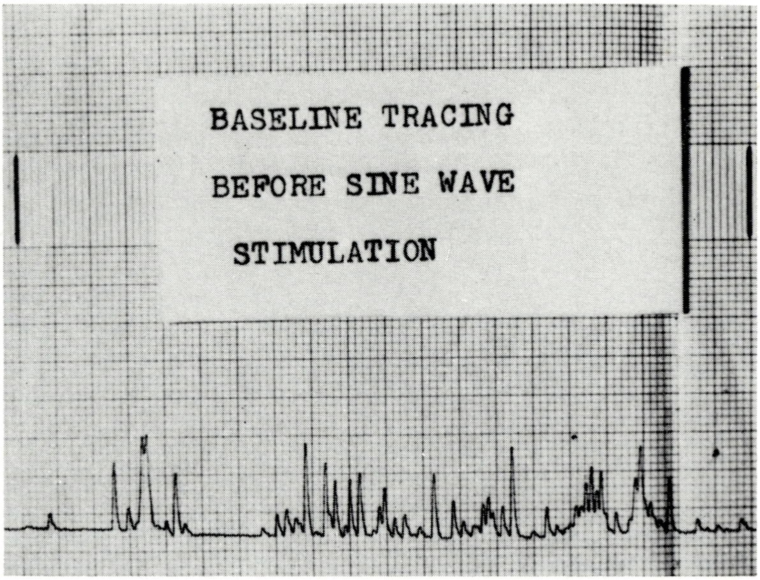

Figure 144: Baseline intestinal motility tracing before acupuncture.

Results:

Two parameters were used to evaluate the intestinal motility 1) the increase in amplitude of the recorded waves; 2) the increase in frequency of waves per 40 second interval in the ACH infused animals, the amplitude

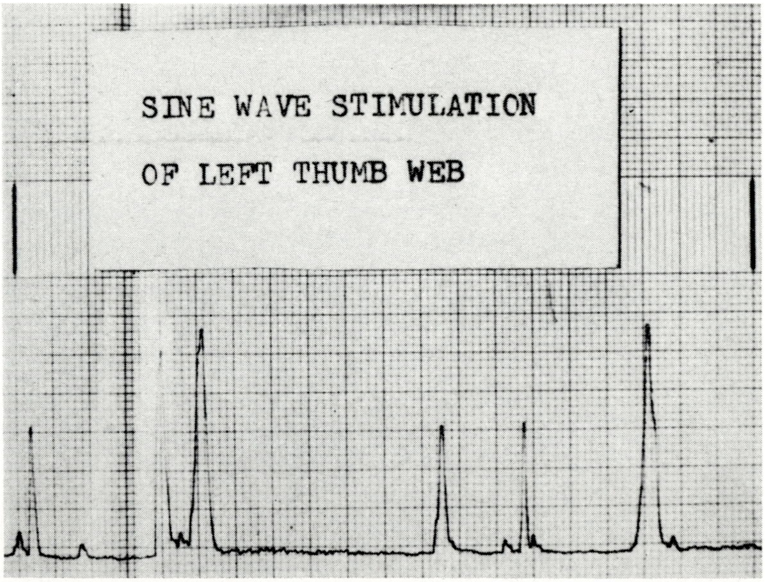

Figure 145: Intestimal mobility tracing after sine wave acupuncture stimulation at the first dorsal web.

reached from 13 to 17 cm H_2O at a rate of three waves per 40 second interval (Figures 142, 143).

In the Sine Wave group the best results were obtained from stimulating either the thumb web or the index web. When the thumb web was stimulated, the amplitude increased from 18 to 28 cm H_2O above baseline at a rate of 3 to 4 contractions per 40 second intervals (Figures 144 and 145). When the index web was stimulated, the amplitude varied from 15 to 21 cm H_2O above baseline at a rate of 2 to 5 contractions per 40 second intervals (Figure 146).

In the delta and square wave groups, the fluctuations of the amplitude rarely exceeded 14 cm above baseline, and the number of contractions per 40 second intervals were quite irregular (Figures 147, 148).

Comments:

The random selection of stimulation points had to be applied since the rabbit, unlike the human species, does not seem to have selective meridian points where the electrical permeability is increased.[11] The areas which give the best results are located near the thumb and index webs which may correspond to the intestinal meridian in humans.[77] Also the best results are obtained with a sine wave of 200 microamperes at a frequency of 10 kilohertz, which is the same wave form, amperage and frequency which gives the best anesthesia results in this laboratory.

The interpretation of wave patterns in the small bowel is difficult. The pre-stimulation wave forms probably represent the segmental and pendular

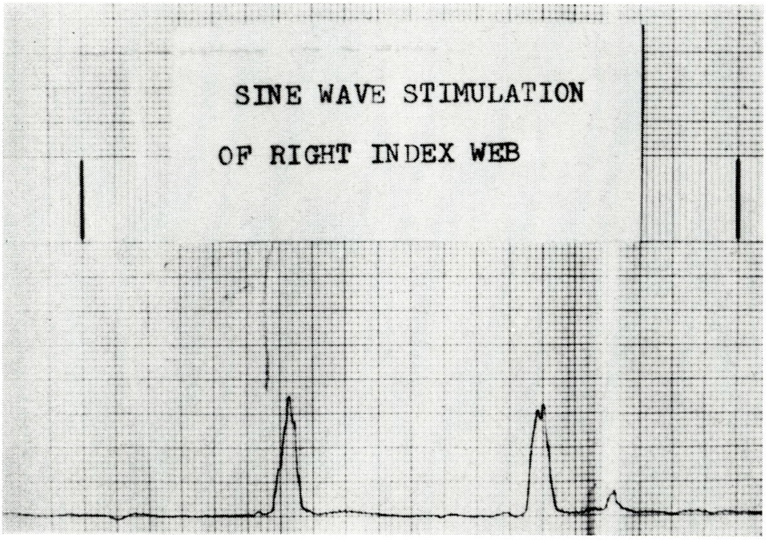

Figure 146: Intestinal motility tracing after sine wave acupuncture stimulation at the index web.

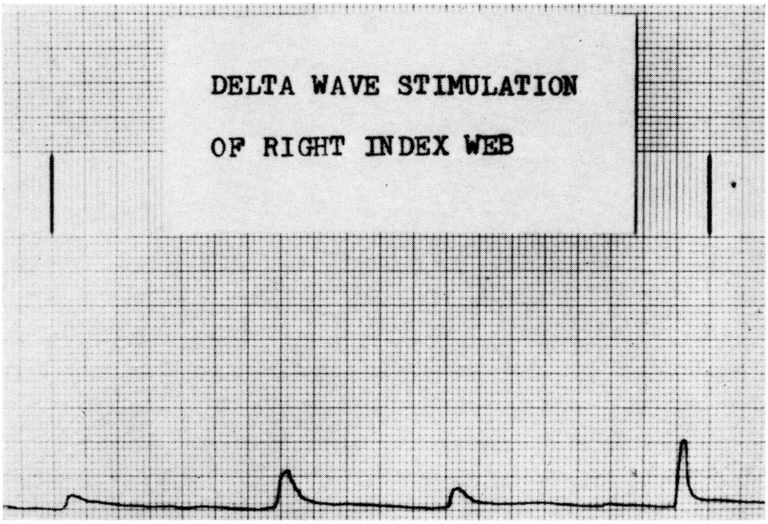

Figure 147: Intestinal motility tracing after Delta wave acupuncture stimulation at the thumb web.

movements of the small bowel which have more to do with mixing the chyme than propelling it, as has been well described in standard physiology texts.[93] The wave forms following acupuncture are similar to those following ACH administration and probably represents peristalsis.

We now plan to study the effect of acupuncture has on vagus nerve output by isolating the vagus nerve and studying the electrical output pre and post acupuncture therapy given at the dorsal webs.

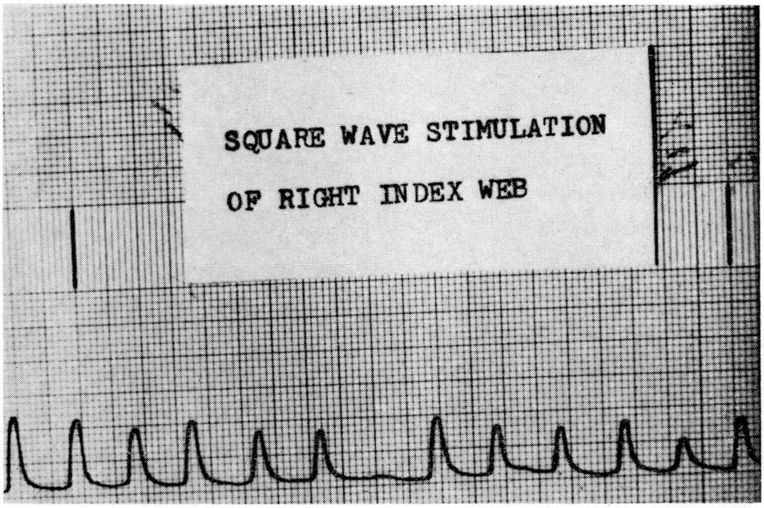

Figure 148: Intestinal motility tracing after square wave acupuncture stimulation at the thumb web.

In summary, albino rabbits have a maximum peristaltic response to acupuncture when given in the form of a sine wave stimulus and applied to the thumb or index web.

SECTION 3: EVALUATION OF ACUPUNCTURE IN CHRONIC PAIN DUE TO OSTEOARTHRITIS

(In Collaboration With Bruce Levy, M.D.)

The efficacy of acupuncture therapy for patients with chronic neck pain due to osteoarthritis has been shown to be statistically significant, using a single and double-blind study technique, in a previous publication by these authors.[94]

This section reports clinical experience with acupuncture used as treatment for patients with chronic neck pain or lower back pain, with or without associated sciatic pain, due to osteoarthritis of the cervical or lumbosacral spines respectively on 108 patients.

Methods of Procedure:

A. Patients:

Studied were a total of 108 reliable adults of both sexes ranging in age from thirty-five to sixty-five years. Fifty-six patients had complaints of neck and shoulder pain due to cervical osteoarthritis and fifty-two patients had complaints of lower back pain, with or without associated sciatic pain, from lumbosacral osteoarthritis. Excluded from the study were patients with mental instability, mutiple complaints not related to their specific diagnosis or those with herniated discs. Business men, hairdressers, housewives, medical technicians, salesmen, and physicians comprised the groups, all of whom were screened carefully for the above indications as well as to ensure that they had no other diseases which could cause similar complaints.

These patients had all been treated by their family physicians and by rheumatologists, neurosurgeons, and/or orthopedic surgeons for more than one year without appreciable improvement, and the majority of them were referred by one of these physicians. Those patients who were not referred, were evaluated by the appropriate specialists at Hahnemann Medical College and Hospital, Philadelphia, Pennsylvania, before acupuncture therapy was begun.

Diagnostic procedure, including careful history taking, range of neck and shoulder or lower back and hip motion, reliable x-rays of cervical spine and shoulder joints or lumbosacral spines and hip joints (myelogram in some patients) and laboratory workup (CBC, SMA-12, coagulation profile, uric acid and urinalysis) had been completed in most of these patients within six months prior to acupuncture treatments. Those patients who had not had some of the studies completed within this prior six month period, had them obtained before beginning treatment. No patient selected in this study had positive physical findings other than osteoarthritis of any of the painful joints.

After being given a careful explanation of the procedure, patients were requested to sign a permit prior to acupuncture. No acupuncture was given on the initial visit, but rather efforts were made to screen the patients to be sure that they would meet study criteria, to evaluate mental stability, to give them a full understanding of the procedure and to emphasize the importance of their assistance in obtaining accurate data.

B. Evaluation Parameters for Improvement:

The first three parameters were of an objective nature and only the last parameter was of a subjective nature.

1. A 50% or greater increase in neck and shoulder or back and hip range of motion as compared to preacupuncture therapy.
2. A 50% or greater decrease in frequency and dosage of medications as compared to preacupuncture therapy.
3. The L-C neurometer readings decreased to 50 microamperes or lower as compared to 100 microamperes or greater acupuncture readings at the tender musculoskeletal arm-shoulder-neck or lumbosacral-sciatic meridian points.
4. Subjective opinion of the patient that his pain was much improved, his ability to perform daily activities was increased, and emotionally the patient felt better.

C. Grouping and Technique:

All patients were treated in the same way, except that those with neck-shoulder pain received their treatment on classic musculoskeletal meridian points listed in Table VIII and those treated with lower back pain, with or without sciatic pain, were treated at the classic points listed in Table IX.

TABLE VIII

POINTS USED FOR TREATMENT OF CERVICAL OSTEOARTHRITIS

Name of Point	*General Body Location*
High Lateral Trapezius	Head and Neck
Para C_1-C_2	Head and Neck
C_7-T_1	Head and Neck
Para C_7-T_1	Head and Neck
Claviculoscapular Junction	Shoulder
Anterior Acromion	Shoulder
Posterior Acromion	Shoulder
Posterior Axillary Crease	Shoulder
Lateral Cubital Crease	Forearm
Dorsal Upper Forearm	Forearm
First Dorsal Metacarpal	Hand
Lateral Fifth Metacarpal	Hand

TABLE IX

POINTS USED FOR TREATMENT OF LUMBOSACRAL OSTEOARTHRITIS

Name of Points	*General Body Location*
Lateral L_2-L_3	Lower Back
Para L_2-L_3	Lower Back
Para L_3-L_4	Lower Back
Para L_4-L_5	Lower Back
Para L_5-S_1	Lower Back
Posterior Trochanter	Gluteal Region
Midgluteal Crease	Gluteal Region
Posterior Midthigh	Thigh
Lateral Upper Tibia	Lower Extremity
Posterior Lateral Malleolus	Ankle

All patients were evaluated by the above four parameters before and after each acupuncture treatment and the results were recorded on the patients chart. If the patient complained of bilateral pain, then at the first treatment the more painful side was treated on successive visits, treatment was given bilaterally at these traditional musculoskeletal meridian acupuncture points.

The acupuncture needle was introduced one centimeter in depth perpendicular to the skin and advanced in various directions until the patient felt an aching, soreness, numbness, or tingling radiation distally or proximally ("Needle Shock"). Each point was treated for two minutes continuously by the manual "sparrow pecking" or twirling motion technique. The same procedure was repeated every three to seven days, at three to ten individual visits on successive visits, if the patient showed positive improvement in all four parameters, had complete disappearance of pain and the neurometer registered zero at all tender points where acupuncture had been given, then no further treatment was given and the patient was discharged.

Results:

The results are tabulated in Tables X and XI. Approximately 80% of the traditional Chinese musculoskeletal meridian acupuncture points for both groups of patients evidenced altered electrical activity of the skin,

TABLE X

EFFECT OF ACUPUNCTURE ON CERVICAL OSTEOARTHRITIS

Group	*Number of Patients*
Total Improvement	14 (25%)
Excellent Improvement	21 (38%)
Satisfactory Improvement	12 (21%)
No Improvement	9 (16%)
Worse	0 (0%)
TOTAL	56 (100%)

TABLE XI

EFFECT OF ACUPUNCTURE ON LUMBOSACRAL OSTEOARTHRITIS

Group	*Number of Patients*
Total Improvement	10 (19%)
Excellent Improvement	19 (37%)
Satisfactory Improvement	14 (27%)
No Improvement	9 (17%)
Worse	0 (0%)
TOTAL	52 (100%)

and these points were always tender by finger pressure. Total improvement meant that the patient had a full range of motion of the diseased joints, was taking no medications, had neurometer readings at zero at all the tender musculoskeletal meridian points, and experienced total subjective improvement. Excellent improvement was evidenced by positive results in all four parameters studied. Those patients with satisfactory improvement had positive results in three out of four of the parameters studied. Patients ranging from no improvement to improvement only in two of the parameters studied were considered not improved. Our criteria for a patient becoming worse after the treatment were a decrease in the range of motion, an increase in the dosage and frequency of medication required, or the subjective opinion of the patient that he or she felt worse as compared to preacupuncture therapy.

Considering both groups of patients together, over 20% had total improvement, and when combining the total and excellent improvement groups, this population of the patients was approximately 60% of the total groups. When the satisfactorily improved groups were added to the above, approximately 83% of the total population or five out of every six patients evidenced a good degree of improvement after acupuncture therapy. These results were statistically significant. Another interesting finding was that no patient became worse after a course of acupuncture therapy.

Discussion:

Oriental reports leave one impressed with the efficacy of acupuncture for the various ailments,[91] but reports of an objective study are lacking. This is our second report of an objective study on the clinical efficacy of acupuncture for osteoarthritis of the spine.[94]

Public demand for acupuncture has been growing while the AMA's stand regarding the practice of acupuncture is neither approval or disapproval. It is therefore absolutely necessary to clarify efficacy in a scientific manner, and it is essential to know whether acupuncture is effective for certain conditions (i.e. postoperative pain, pain from carcinoma, impotence, Tic Douloureaux, etc.).

Scientific speculation among physicians has been reported. Doctor Kroger[88] in a letter to the editor (JAMA) pointed out that acupuncture is a form of hyponosis. Others believe the efficacy of acupuncture could be explained by the concept of the Gate Control Theory of pain or its modification speculating the existence of inhibitory gates located in the internuncial pool of the spinal cord and the thalamus.[4]

The mechanism of action of acupuncture is not fully understood at this time. Traditional explanations of the five element theory and the positive and negative forces concept prevented scientific explanation for a long period of time. At present, explanations of the mechanisms of acupuncture are speculative and based primarily on neurophysiological data. Some consider acupuncture a mode of hypnosis. However, the fact that acupuncture does work in animals has been shown in our laboratory. We know from our laboratory work (Chapter 6; Section 1) that acupuncture is mediated through the nervous system, requires an intact, functioning nervous system to be successful and some contact with the central nervous system is necessary for acupuncture analgesia to be maximally successful. We also found that acupuncture stimulation of the muscle, tendon or bone would not produce analgesia, while stimulation of the nerve itself would produce analgesia, in addition, our clinical experiments mitigate against the concept that acupuncture is a form of hypnosis.

Our clinical study indicates that 80% of the traditional acupuncture points used in this study are actually points where electrical activity of the skin is significantly altered. From our laboratory research, we speculate that these points are those where somatic nerve branches run relatively superficially. Japanese investigators[1] accept the points where electrical activity of the skin is altered as acupuncture points and name them as "Ryodo Ketsu (Electrically permeable point).

An L-C neurometer (Figure 36) was used to determine altered electrical activity and this was defined as having a neurometer reading at the specific point of 100 microamperes or greater. Those points with these readings were always tender to palpation. The negative arm of the neurometer was held in the patient's left hand, and he or she was instructed to grip it as hard as possible. The positive, detecting arm was fitted with a spring so that a constant pressure was always applied to all the points irregardless of examiner or patient.

Modern medicine as developed in the western hemisphere and now practiced throughout the world appears to be highly effective in the cure of disease. However, there are still certain syndromes and diseases for which modern medicine is not indicated or ever effective. Chronic pain is certainly one of them and frequently becomes a problem for the patient himself, then the family and even the nation. The patients suffering from chronic pain due to osteoarthritis are considerable in number, and they may be helped by properly conducted acupuncture. It is essential, that these patients be throughly evaluated medically in order not to lose the golden period during which an underlying disorder could possibly be treated effectively by standard modern medical therapy.

Summary:

Over 80% of the traditional musculoskeletal meridian points used in this study showed altered electrical activity and were tender to palpation. Ninety of the 108 patients (83%) in this study showed objective and subjective, satisfactory improvement after acupuncture therapy. Acupuncture has a statistically significant efficacy in the treatment of chronic pain resulting from osteoarthritis of the cervical or lumbosacral spines.

REFERENCES

1. Hiyodo, M.: *New Management of Pain.* Tokyo, Chiyugai Igakushiya, 1970.
2. Judovich, B., Bates, W.: *Pain Syndromes.* Philadelphia, Davis Co, 1953.
3. Takahashi, K.: *Recognition of Chinese Medicine.* Tokyo, NHK Publisher, 1969.
4. Melzack, R., Wall, P. D.: Pain mechanisms: a new theory. *Science,* 150:971-979, 1965.
5. Diamond, E. G.: Acupuncture anesthesia. *JAMA, 218*:1558, 1971.
6. Fulton, J. F.: *A Textbook of Physiology.* Philadelphia, Saunders, 1955.
7. NIH Ad Hoc Committee on Acupuncture. *Acupuncture Research Conference.* NIH, Bethesda, Feb 28 and March 1, 1973.
8. Chu, Lien: *Hsin chen-chiu hsueh (Textbook of Modern Acupuncture and Moxibustion).* The People's Hygiene Publishing House, Peking, 1957.
9. Veith, I.: *Huang ti nei ching su wen (The Yellow Emperor's Classic of Internal Medicine).* University of California Press, Berkeley, 1966.
10. Takahashi, K.: *Recognition of Chinese Medicine.* NHK Publisher, Tokyo, 1969.
11. Nakaya, Y.: *Practice of Electropermeable Points.* Riyodoraky Kenkyushiyo, Tokyo, 1965.
12. Hiyodo, M.: *New Management of Pain.* Chiyugai Igakushiya, Tokyo, 1970.
13. Serizawa, K.: *Science of Acupuncture.* Iyaky Shiyuppan, Tokyo, 1959.
14. Takahashi, K.: *Study of Theory in Acupunture.* Harikyu, Tokyo, 13:45, 1964.
15. Yabudchi, K.: *Ancient Science in China.* Kadokawa Shiyoten, Tokyo, 1964.
16. Serizawa, K.: *Study of Meridian Points.* Gomashiyobo, Tokyo, 1971.
17. Serizawa, K.: *Medical Study of Meridian Points and Lines.* Nihon Onkyushi, Tokyo, *24*:389, 1960.
18. Infectious Disease, July 3, 1971.
19. Diamond, E. G.: Acupuncture anesthesia. *JAMA,* Vol. *218,* No. 10:1558-1563, December 6, 1971.
20. Wulfsohn, N. L., and Saules, A.: *The Nervous System and Electric Currents.* (Proceedings of the 4th Annual National of the Neuroelectric Society, held in San Antonio, Texas, March 10-12, 1971), Plenum Press, New York, 1971.
21. Limoge, A.: Obstetric electro-analgesia. In Wulfsohn, N. L., and Saules, A. (Eds.): *The Nervous System and Electric Currents.* Plenum, New York, 1971.
22. Negovski, A. A., Kuzin, M. N., and Liuentseu, B. J.: Electro-anesthesia for electrical cardioversion. In Wulfsohn, N. L., and Saules, A. (Eds.): *The Nervous System and Electric Currents.* Plenum, New York, 1971.
23. Zuperku, E. J., Saules, A., Larson, S. J.: Rectangular electro-anesthesia currents and the primary visual pathways. In Wulfsohn, N. L., and Saules, A.: *The Nervous System and Electric Currents.* Plenum, New York, 1971.
24. Larson, S. J., and Saules, A.: Physiologic effects of electro-anesthesia. *Surgery, 64*:281, 1968.
25. Saules, A., and Larson, S. J.: Electro-anesthesia research. In Clynes and Milsum: *Biomedical Engineering Systems.* New York, McGraw Hill, 1970.
26. Saules, A., and Larson, S. J.: Physiological mechanisms related to electro-anesthesia. In Musacchia and Saunders: *Depressed Metabolism.* New York, Elsevier, 1969.

27. Winkler, E. R., Stratton, D. B., and Rubin, M.: Electro-anesthesia: by a new portable battery powered device. In Wulfsohn, N. L., and Saules, A. (Eds.): *The Nervous System and Electric Currents.* Plenum, 1971.
28. Hause, L. L.: *Electrophysiological Effects of Electric Fields on the Individual Neuron As Studied by Mathematical Modeling and Bioelcetri Methods.* Marquette University, Wisconsin, 1970.
29. Siegesmud, K. A., Saules, A., and Larson, S. J.: Effects of electro-anesthesia on synaptic ultrastructure. *Neurological Science, 9*:89, 1969.
30 Toleikis, J. R.: *Effects of Electro-anesthesia Upon Cerebral Unit Potentials.* Proceedings of the 2nd International Symposium on Electrosleep and electro-anesthesia. Graz, Austria, 1969.
31. Limoge, A.: Mechanism of electro-analgesia. In Wulfsohn, N. L., and Saules, A. (Eds.): *The Nervous System and Electric Currents.* Plenum, New York, 1971.
32. Reigel, D. H., Saules, A., and Larson, S. J.: Effects of Electro-anesthesia upon circulatory serontonin. In Wulfsohn, N. L., and Saules, A (Eds.): *The Nervous System and Electric Currents.* Plenum, New York, 1971.
33. Jouvet, M.: Biogenic amines and the states of sleep. *Science, 163*:32, 1969.
34. Pozos, R. S., Richardson, A. W., and Kaplan, H. M.: Mode of production and locus of action of electro-anesthesia in dogs. *Anesth Analg, 48*:341, 1969.
35. Dallman, D. E., Reigel, D. H., Zilber, S., and Saules, A.: A new electrode holder for experimental electro-anesthesia. *Med Biol Eng, 17*:449, 1969.
36. Reigel, D. H., Saules, A., and Larson, S. J.: Surgical experiences with electro-anesthesia. In Wulfsohn, N. L., and Saules, A. (Eds.): *The Nervous System and Electric Currents.* Plenum, New York, 1971.
37. Reigel, D. H., Larson, S. J., Saules, A., Christman, N. T., Dallman, D. E., and Heuschel, E. O.: Abdominal surgery under electro-anesthesia. Abstracts of the Neuro-electric Conference, *5*:27, 1969.
38. Beecher, H. K.: *Management of Subjective Responses.* Oxford University Press, New York, 1959.
39. Palos, S.: *The Chinese Art of Healing.* Herder and Herder, New York, 1971.
41. Wu, Wei-ping.: *Formulaire d'acupuncture.* Paris, 1959. Dec. 21, 1958.
41. Wu Wei-ping.: *Formulaire d'acupuncture.* Paris, 1959.
42. Nanking Chinese Medical School: *Outline of Chinese Medicine.* Iyakueisei Shiyuppanshiya, Hong Kong, 1969.
43. Croizier, R. C.: *Traditional Medicine in Modern China.* Harvard University Press, Berkeley and Los Angeles, 1966.
44. Chinese Peoples Air Force Shinyo Hospital: *Rapid Needle Therapy.* Peoples Health Publisher, 1969.
45. Kaizuka, S.: *History of World.* Chiyuwokoronshiya, Tokyo, 1902.
46. Judovich, B. D., and Bates, W.: *Pain Syndrome.* Philadelphia, Davis Co, 1953,
47. Mann, P. L., and Chen, C. H.: Mechanism of acupuncture anesthesia (the two gate control theory). *Dis Nerv Sys, 33*:730, 1972.
48. Liu, T.: Introducing experience of using acupuncture to treat goiter. *Journal of Chinese Traditional Medicine.* No. 6-1960, 2223, June 5, 1960.
49. Honma, Y.: *Meridian Points.* Idonoihonsiya, Tokyo, 1957.

50. Nakaya, Y.: *Treatment by Electropermeable Points.* Riyodoraku Kenkyushiyo, Tokyo, 1965.
51. Nakaya, Y.: *Outline Electropermeability in Medicine.* Riyodoraky Kenkyushiyo, Tokyo, 1968.
52. Nagahama, Y.: *New Study of Acupuncture. Sogenshiya,* Tokyo, 1964.
53. Akaba, K.: *Subcutaneous Needling.* Idonoihonsiya, Tokyo, 1966.
54. Nagahama, Y.: *Outline of Oriental and Western Medicine.* Sogenshiya, Tokyo, 1961.
55. Kinoshita, H.: *Outline of Acupuncture.* Nichonchiyaw School of Acupuncture, Tokyo, 1959.
56. *Current Acupuncture in Japan.* Idononihmyshiya, Tokyo, 1969.
57. Veith, I.: *Huang ti nei ching su wen (The Yellow Emperor's Classic of Internal Medicine)* (new edition). University of California Press, Berkeley and Los Angeles, 1966.
58. Huard, P., and Wong, M.: *Chinese Medicine.* McGraw-Hill, New York, Toronto, 1968.
59. Mann, F.: *Acupuncture, the Ancient Chinese Art of Healing,* 2nd ed. William Heineman Medical Books Ltd., London, 1971.
60. Liang, Ch'iu: Introduction of a new spot "ya-t'ung-ling" in acupuncture for treating toothache. *Chiang-su Chung-i (Kiangsu Chinese Traditional Medicine),* 1966.
61. Chang, T.: Discussion of the Application of Acupuncture at the ho-ku Site. *Chiang-su Chung-i (Kiangsu Chinese Traditional Medicine),* 1966.
63. Jen, S., and Chao, C. C.: Acupuncture in the treatment of pharyngeal paralysis: report of 22 cases. *Shan-tung I-k'an* (Shantung Medical Journal), 1964.
64. Li, Ching-chow and Chin, ch'in: Efficacy observations in acupunctural treatment of acute jaundicial, infectious hepatitis." *Shanghai Chung-i Tsa-chih (Shanghai Journal of Chinese Traditional Medicine),* 1965.
65. *Chung I Tsa-chih (Journal of Chinese Traditional Medicine),* Peking, 1964.
66. Initial clinical observations in acupunctural prevention and treatment of epidemic influenza in 1,000 cases. Anonymous: *Chung-i Tsa-chih (Journal of Chinese Traditional Medicine),* 1964.
67. Tobimatsu, G., and Kobayashi, A.: Chinese acupuncture and practice. *Nihonijishinpo, 2523*:29, 1972.
68. Suzuki, F., and Tobimatsu, G.: Chinese acupuncture anesthesia. *Nihonijishinpo, 2521*:3, 1972.
69. Acupuncture Anesthesia Apparatus, Portable Type (Model 71-7) The Peoples' Republic of China.
70. Limoge A.: Electric Anesthesia. Proceedings of the 4th Annual National Conference of the Neuroelectric Society, San Antonio, Texas, March 10-12, 1971.
71. Negovski, B. A., Kuzin, M. N., Liventsev, H. M., Tabak, B. J., Gurvich, H. L., Zhukovskii, V. D., Cherviakov, M. E., and Kaverina, K. P.: *Electro-Anesthesia for Electrical Cardioversion.* Proceedings of the 4th Annual National Conference of the Neurolectric Socitey, San Antonio, Texas, March 10-12, 1971.
72. Winkler, E. R., Stratton, M. A., Rubin, M., and Richardson, A. W.: *Electroanesthesia by a New Portable Battery Powered Device.* Proceedings of

the 4th Annual National Conference of the Neuroelectric Society, San Antonio, Texas, March 10-12, 1971.
73. Reigel, H. D., Sances, A., Larson, S. J., and Hoffman, N.: Effect of Electroanesthesia Upon Circulating Serotonin. Proceedings of the 4th Annual National Conference of the Neuroelectric Society, San Antonio, Texas, March 10-12, 1971.
74. Reigel, D. H., Sances, A., and Larson, S. J.: Surgical Annual National Conference of the Neuroelectric Society, San Antonio, Texas, March 10-12, 1971.
75. Personal Communication.
76. Klemm, W. R.: *Animal Electroencephalography,* Academic Press, 1969.
77. Mann, Felix, *Acupuncture.* New York, Vintage, 1972.
78. Wall, R. and Sweet, W. H.: Temporary abolition of pain in man. *Science, 155*:108-109, 1967.
79. Man, P. L., and Chen, C. H.: Acupuncture anesthesia, a new theory and clinical study. *Current Therapeutic Research, 14*:7, July, 1972.
80. Matsumoto, T.: Evaluation of acupuncture in management of gastrointestinal atony. *Surg Forum, 23*:401, 1972.
81. Kelly, K. A., and Code, C. F.: Effect of transthroacic vagotomy on canine gastric electrical activity. *Gastroenterology, 57*:51, 1969.
82. Kelly, K. A.: Gastric motility and ulcer surgery. *Surg Clin N Amer, 51*:927, 1972.
83. Forbes, T. W.: Problems in measurement of electrodermal phenomena. *Psychophysiology, 1*:26, 1964.
84. Edelberg, R., and Wright, D. J.: Two galvanic skin response effector organs and their stimulus specificity. *Psychophysiology, 1*:39, 1964.
85. Neumann, E.: The early history of electrodermal research. *Psychophysiology, 6*:39, 1970.
86. People's Republic of China Air Force Hospital at Shinyan, *Quick Needle Therapy.* People's Health Publisher, Tokyo, 1969.
87. Matsumoto, T., and Hayes, M.: Acupuncture electric phenomenon of the skin and postvagotomy gastrointestinal atony. *Am J Surg, 125, 176*:180, 1973.
88. Kroger, W. S.: Hyponosis and acupuncture. *JAMA, 220*:1012, 1972.
89. Matsumoto, T.: Acupuncture and U.S. medicine. *JAMA, 220*:1010, May, 1972.
90. Plum, F. and Posner, J.B.: Diagnosis of Stupor and Coma. F.A. Davis Company, Philadelphia, Pa.
91. Geiger, H. J.: How acupuncture anesthetizes—a Chinese explanation. *Medical World News, Vol. 14,* No. 27, pp. 51-61, July 13, 1973.
92. Bass, P., and Weisbrodt, N. W.: Current Concepts on Pharmacology of Gastrointestinal Motility. Gastrointestinal Motility—International Symposium, Academic Press, New York and London pp. 149-167, 1969.
93. Physiology and Biophysics—Ruch and Patton, 19th Edition Chapter 48, Movements of Small Intestine. W.B. Saunders Company, Philadelphia, and London, 1965.
94 Matsumoto, T., Levy, B., and Ambruso, V.: Clinical Evaluation of Acupuncture. Amer. Surgeon (to be published).

APPENDIX I

Acupuncture Points (English Terms)

Anterior acromion, 42, 62, 64-65, 80, 187
Anterior lower fibula, 44, 71, 77, 78, 81
Anterior upper fibula, 44, 68, 69, 75, 76, 78, 80, 81, 84, 92, 145

C_1-C_2, 42, 50-51, 76, 79, 85
C_7-T_1, 42, 53, 76, 148, 187
Claviculoscapular junction, 44, 64, 80, 187

Dorsal distal forearm, 43, 61, 75, 77, 79, 80, 85
Dorsal low forearm, 43, 61, 62, 80, 82,
Dorsal upper forearm, 43, 61, 62, 79-80, 92, 187

Fifth lateral metacarpal, 43, 61, 74, 76, 77, 80, 85-86, 187
Finger tip, 43, 63-64, 80
First dorsal web, 43, 60, 72, 74-87, 92, 187
First metatarsal, 44, 70-71, 81
Fourth dorsal web, 43, 60, 61, 75, 80, 92

Glabella, 42, 45-46, 76, 79, 87, 92

High lateral trapezius, 42, 50, 74, 76, 77, 79, 84-88, 92, 140, 147

Inferior masseter, 42, 46, 76, 68, 92
Inframastoid, 42, 49, 76, 87, 88, 92, 140, 147
Infranasal, 35, 42, 48-49, 76, 85
Infratemporal, 42, 46, 76, 78, 82, 140, 147
Inter M.P. joint, 43, 63

Lateral cubital crease, 43, 62, 65, 72, 74, 75, 77, 80-86, 92, 187
Lateral infraorbital, 42, 47, 48, 87, 88
Lateral inguinal, 43, 55, 56, 78
Lateral L_2-L_3, 43, 56, 57, 59, 79, 149, 188
Lateral midthigh, 44, 67, 81
Lateral oral angle, 42, 49, 76, 92
Lateral thyroid, 42, 51, 76, 82, 86
Lateral umbilicus, 43, 55, 78, 82, 83
Lateral upper tibia, 35, 44, 67-69, 72, 74, 76-86, 92, 145, 150
Low hypogastrium, 43, 55, 78, 84-85

Median canthus, 42, 46, 47, 76, 87, 88
Median popliteal crease, 44, 71, 73, 81
Median supra patella, 44, 71, 73, 81
Midepigastrium, 43, 54, 78, 80-83
Mid-eyebrow, 42, 45-46, 76, 140
Mid-gastrocnemius, 44, 69-70, 77, 81
Midgluteal crease, 44, 65, 66, 81, 144, 150, 188
Midinfraorbital, 42, 47, 76, 88
Midlateral humerus, 44, 64, 65, 80
Midsternum, 43, 53, 78

Para C_1-C_2, 42, 50, 51, 187
Para C_7-T_1, 42, 52-53, 82, 143, 187
Para L_2-L_3, 43, 56-58, 77, 79, 84, 143, 149, 188
Para L_4-L_5, 43, 56-57, 59, 79, 143, 188

Para L_5-S_1, 43, 56, 57, 59, 79, 87, 143, 188
Para S_1-S_2, 43, 56, 57, 59, 79, 143
Para S_2-S_3, 43, 56, 57, 59, 79, 143
Para T_2-T_3, 43, 56, 57, 79, 143
Para T_3-T_4, 43, 56, 57, 79, 143, 148
Para T_5-T_6, 43, 56, 57, 58, 79, 80, 143, 148
Para T_7-T_8, 43, 56, 57, 58, 79, 80, 84, 143, 148
Para T_9-T_{10}, 43, 56, 57, 58, 79, 143, 148
Para T_{10}-T_{11}, 43, 56, 57, 58, 79, 143, 149
Para T_{11}-T_{12}, 43, 56, 57, 58, 79, 82, 143, 149
Para T_{12}-L_1, 43, 56, 57, 58, 79, 83, 143, 149
Posterior acromion, 44, 62, 64, 80, 187
Posterior anal, 43, 56, 57, 59, 79, 143
Posterior axillary crease, 44, 64, 65, 80, 187
Posterior earlobe, 42, 48, 49, 76, 86
Posterior lateral malleolus, 44, 70, 71, 73, 74, 77, 78, 81, 84, 188
Posterior low tibia, 44, 69, 70, 81, 83, 84, 85, 92
Posterior medial malleolus, 44, 70, 71, 75, 81
Posterior midthigh, 44, 66, 67, 73, 74, 81, 146, 150, 188
Posterior trochanter, 44, 64, 66, 75, 76, 77, 81, 188

Radial styloid process, 43, 62, 80

Sole of foot, 44, 70, 73, 81
Sub breast, 43, 54, 78
Subxyphoid, 43, 53, 54, 78
Superior tragus, 42, 47, 48, 76, 186
Supraorbital, 42, 44, 45, 76, 92
Suprapubic, 43, 55, 56, 78
Suprasternal, 42, 51, 52, 53, 76, 81, 82, 83, 86

Temporal, 42, 45, 76, 79, 80, 92
T_3-T_4, 43, 56, 59, 79, 80

Upper hypogastrium, 43, 55, 78
Upper posterior tibia, 44

Vertex, 42, 44, 75, 76
Volar distal forearm, 43, 63, 72, 74, 80, 82, 83, 84, 85, 86, 92

APPENDIX II

Acupuncture Points (Oriental Terms)

Japanese	*Chinese*	*Meridian Notation*	*Page*
Amon	Ya-Men	GV 15	42, 50, 51, 76, 79, 85
Ashi-Sanri	Tsu-San-Li	S 36	35, 44, 67, 68, 69, 72, 74, 76-79, 81-86, 92, 145, 150, 188
Bichiyu	Chien		42, 45, 46, 76, 140
Bokoyu	P'ang-K'uang-Yu	B 28	43, 56, 57, 59, 79, 143
Chiso	Ti-Chang	S 7	42, 49, 76, 92, 45, 52, 53, 82, 143, 187
Chyokyo	Ch'ang-Ch'iang	GV 1	43, 56, 57, 59, 78, 143
Chyukan	Chung-Wuan	CV 12	43, 54, 78, 80, 81, 83
Chyukyoku	Chung-Chi	CV 3	53, 55, 78, 84, 85
Chyushyo	Chung-Chu	T_3	43, 60, 61, 75, 80, 92
Daichyoyu	Ta-Chang-Yu	B 25	43, 56, 57, 59, 79, 143, 188
Daizui	Ta-Ch'ui	GV 14	42, 53, 76, 148, 187
Danchyu	Shan-Chung	CV 17	43, 53, 78
Eifu	Yi-Fong	T 17	42, 48, 49, 76, 86
Fuchi	Feng-Shih	GB 31	42, 50, 74, 76, 77, 79
Fuichi	Fong-Chih	GB 20	44, 67, 81
Fumon	Feng-Men	B 12	43, 56, 57, 79, 143
Gaikan	Wai-Kuah	T 5	43, 61, 75, 77, 79, 80, 85
Gekan	Hsia-Kuan	S 2	42, 46, 76, 78, 92, 140, 147
Gokoku	Ho-ku	LI 4	43, 60, 72, 74-76, 78, 80-87, 92, 187
Hachija	Pa-Hsieh	— —	43, 63
Haiyu	Fei-Yu	B 13	43, 56, 57, 79, 143, 148
Hiyu	P'i-yu	B 20	43, 56-68, 79, 82, 143, 149
Hyankue	Pai-Hui	GV 20	42, 44, 75, 76
Iho	— — —	— —	43, 55, 56, 78
Imei	I-Ming	— —	42, 49, 76, 87, 88, 92, 140, 147
Indo	Yin-Tang	— —	42, 45, 46, 76, 79, 87, 92
Inryosen	Yin-Lin-Ch'uan	SP 9	44
Iyu	Wei-Yu	B 21	43, 56-58, 79, 83, 143, 149
Jimon	Erh-Men	T 21	42, 47, 48, 76, 86
Jinchiyu	Jen-Chung	GV 26	35, 42, 48, 49, 76, 85
Jingei	Jen-Ying	S 9	42, 51, 76, 82, 86
Jinyu	Shen-yu	B 23	43, 56-58, 77, 79, 84, 143, 149, 188
Jissen	Shih-Hsuan	— —	43, 63, 64, 80
Kakuyu	Ke-Yu	B 17	43, 56, 58, 79, 80, 84, 143, 148
Kanchyo	Huan-Tiao	GB 30	44, 64, 66, 75-77, 81, 188
Kangen	Kuan-Yuan	CV 4	43, 55, 78, 81-84, 87, 92
Kangenyu	Kuan-Yuan-Yu	B 26	43, 56, 57, 59, 79, 87, 143, 188
Kanyu	Kenye	B 18	43, 56-68, 79, 143, 148
Kengu	Chien-Yu	LI 15	44, 62, 64, 65, 80, 187
Kenko	Chien-Liao	T 14	44, 62, 64, 80, 187
Kentei	Chien-Chen	SI 9	44, 64, 65, 80, 187
Ketsukai	Hsueh-Hai	SP 10	44, 71, 73, 81

Japanese	*Chinese*	*Meridian Notation*	*Page*
Kikai	Chi-Hai	CV 6	43, 55, 78
Kokei	Hou-chi	SI 3	43, 61, 74, 76, 77, 80, 85, 86, 187
Konron	Kun-Chun	B 60	44, 70, 71, 73, 74, 77, 78, 81, 84, 188
Kyokotsu	Chu-ku	LI 16	44, 64, 80, 187
Kyoku Kotsu	Chu-ku	CV 2	43, 55, 56, 78
Kyokuchi	Chu-Ch'ih	LI 11	43, 62, 65, 72, 74, 75, 77, 80, 81, 83-86, 92, 187
Kyokusen	Chu-Chuan	LV 8	44, 71, 73, 81
Kyoshiya	Chia-Che	S 3	42, 46, 76, 78, 92
Kyubi	Chiu-Wei	CV 15	43, 53, 54, 78
Kyugo	Chiu-Hon		42, 47, 48, 87, 88
Letsuketsu	Lieh-Ch'ueh	L 7	43, 62, 80
Mumei			43, 56, 59, 79, 80
Naikan	Nei-Kuan	P 6	43, 63, 72, 74, 80, 82-86, 92
Nyukon	Ju-Ken	S 18	43, 54, 78
	Pi-Nao	LI 14	44, 64, 65, 80
Saninko	San-Yin-Chiao	SP 6	44, 69, 70, 81, 83-85, 92
Seimei	Ching-Ming	B 1	42, 46, 47, 76, 87, 88
Shiko	Chih-Kou	T 6	43, 61, 62, 80, 82
Shinyu	Hsin-Yu	B 15	43, 56-58, 79, 80, 143, 148
Shishitsu	Chih-Shih	B 47	43, 56, 57, 59, 79, 149, 188
Shitoku	Szu-Tu	T 9	43, 61, 62, 79, 80, 92, 187
Shiyofu	Chung-Fu	B 50	44, 65, 66, 81, 144, 150, 188
Shiyokyu	Cheng-Chi	S 4	42, 47, 76, 88
Shyochyoyu	Hsiao-Chang-Yu	B 27	43, 56, 57, 59, 79, 143
Shyozan	Cheng-Shan	B 57	44, 69, 70, 77, 81
Tanyu	Tanyu	B 19	43, 56-58, 79, 143, 149
Taikei	tai-Chi	K 3	44, 70, 71, 75, 181
Taishiyo	T'ai-ch'ung	LV 3	44, 70, 71, 81
Taiyo	Tai-Yang		42, 45, 76, 79, 80, 92
Tenchyu	Tien-Chu	B 10	42, 50-51, 187
Tensu	T'ien-shu	S 25	43, 55, 178, 82-83
Tentotsu	T'ien-T'u	CV 22	42, 51-53, 76, 81-83, 86
Yinmon	Yin-men	B 51	44, 66, 67, 73, 74, 81, 146, 150, 188
Yohaku	Yang-Pei	GB 14	42, 44, 45, 76, 92
Yoryosen	Yang-Lin-Chuan	GB 34	44, 68, 69, 75, 76, 78, 80, 81, 84, 92, 145, 150
Yosen	Yung-Ch'uan	K 1	44, 70, 73, 81
Zetsukotsu	Chueh-ku		44, 71, 77, 78, 81

INDEX

A

Abdominal distention, 54
Abdominal pain, 49, 54, 55
Acetylcholine, 13, 181, 182, 184
ACH administration, 184
Acupuncture anesthesia, 11, 89-91, 165-167
  advantages of acupuncture anesthesia, 89-90
  disadvantages of acupuncture anesthesia, 90
Acupuncture duration, 34
Acupuncture intervals, 34
Acupuncture needle holder, 30
Acupuncture needles, 11
Acupuncture points, 40
Acupuncture Points (English), 196
Acupuncture Points (Oriental), 198
A delta fiber, 21
Ad Hoc committee of NIH recommendations, 151-152
Alpha fiber, 21
Alpha rhythm, 176-178
Amperage, 103
Analgesia, 129, 176
Analgesic patters with acupuncture, 173-179
Anemia, 85, 149
Angina, 54, 139
Angina pectoris, 49, 54, 58, 63
Ankle pain, 78
Anoxia, 58
Arm pain, 62
Arm paralysis, 63, 84-85
Arrythmia, 139
Arterial blood pressure, 99
Asthma, 53, 54, 56, 58, 82, 139, 148
Auricular fibrillation, 109
Autonomic nervous system, 19-21

B

Backache, 49, 52, 56, 58-59, 61, 65-67, 71, 74, 77, 148-150
Bacteriologic study, 97
Basic clinical knowledge, 23-24
Beta fiber, 21
Beta rhythm, 176-178
Bilateral chest pain, 69
Biliary system diseases, 58
Blindness, 50
Blocking points, 139
Blood pressure, 113
Bon Han fluid, 19
Bon Han granules, 19
Brady kinin, 13
Brain stem, 14
Bronchitis, 56

C

Calf pain, 70
Carcinoma, 189
Cardiac asthma, 58
Cardiospasm, 139
Cardioversion, 109
Carrageenin inflammed paws, 101
Casual factor, 12
Cataracts, 87
Cathodal level, 112
Cervical spine, 186, 191
C fibers, 21
Chest pain, 63, 69, 80, 139, 148
China Acupuncture Anesthesia apparatus, 71-1, 94-96, 151-152, 172-173, 177
Chinese medicine, 3, 11, 17
Cholelithiasis, 139
Chordotomy, 13
Chronic pain states, 138, 152
Chyme, 184
Cingulotomy, 13
Circulatory insufficiency, 139
Circulatory serotonin, 111
Coagulation profile, 186
Cold, 52, 54, 82
Colic pain, 58
Colitis, 58-59, 149-150
Complications, 35
Conjunctivitis, 46-47
Consicousness, 177
Consent form, 152-154
Constipation, 54-55, 62, 82-83, 148
Consultants' reports, 156-161
Contact method, 32
Convulsions, 61, 85
Cortex, 121
Cough, 53, 56, 62, 147-148
Current, 104
Cutaneous anesthesia, 122
Cycles, 106

D

DC current, 9, 11, 112
Deafness, 47, 49, 60-61, 63, 85-86
Delta wave, 105-106, 108, 110, 171, 181, 183-184
Dental pain, 46, 49, 60-61, 64, 78-79
Diabetes, 49, 58, 71, 149
Diabetes mellitus, 71
Diarrhea, 54, 55
Dizziness, 35, 46, 50, 73, 147

Dorsal column stimulation, 13
Dorsal horn, 121
Double blind study, 134-138
Dysmenorrhea, 59, 68, 70-71, 87
Dyspnea, 52, 54, 56, 63, 148
Dysuria, 68, 70, 73, 85

E

Ear disorders, 47
Ear needles, 93
Eczema, 62, 73, 186
Edema of face, 49
Edemogen, 101
EEG, 99, 102-104, 106-108, 111, 130-131, 176-177, 179
EKG, 99
Elbow pain, 77, 147
Electric acupuncture, 6-12, 33-34, 94-96, 111, 116-121, 134
Electricity on the meridian, 12
Electric current, 11
Electric energy, 9, 11
Electric permeability, 12, 124
Electric potential, 20
Electric resistance, 6
Electric units, 12
Electrical activity, 191
Electrical cardioversion, 109
Electrical polarization, 11
Electroanesthesia, 109
Electrocardiogram, 113
Electroencephalogram, 102
Electropermeability, 42
Electropermeable line, 20
Electropermeable points, 20
Electropermissive phenomena, 20
EMG artifact, 113
Enuresis, 84
Epilepsy, 52
Evaluation forms, 154-161
Evoked potential, 111
Experimentally induced joint inflammation, 101
Eye disorders, 46-47, 51, 61, 147
Eye pain, dizziness, 46
Eye signs, 113

F

Facial edema, 49
Facial paralysis, 45, 46, 49
Facial tremor, 61
Fever, 52
Finger numbness, 63
Finger pain, 61, 63
Finger pressure, 94
Five elements, 17
Floating pulse, 17
Foot joint pain, 71
Forearm pain, 62
Fracture of rib, 139
Fracture of spine, 139
Free-hand method, 26
Frontal headache, 45-46

G

Gallbladder, 58, 149
Galovanic device, 10, 133
Gas analysis method, 127
Gastric atony, 83-84, 122-129
Gastric disorders, 58
Gastric emptying, 127
Gastric pain, 139
Gastric stasis, 127
Gastritis, 58, 148
Gastroelectrical activity, 121
Gastrointestinal disorders, 58
Gastropathophysiology, 128
Gate control theory, 21, 121
General anesthesia, 11
Glaucoma, 47, 87
Goiter, 51
GU disorders, 55, 71
Gynecological disorders, 55, 149-150

H

H+, 13
Habitual constipation, 62
Hahnemann Medical College & Hospital, 138
Hand motion, 94
Headache, 45-46, 51, 53, 61-62, 71, 73, 79-80, 147
Heart disease, 54, 58, 147-148
Heart pain, 49
Hematemesis, 63
Hemiplegia, 62, 65, 68, 69, 71, 149
Hemorrhoids, 60, 66
Hepatitis, 58, 148-149
Herpes zoster, 139
Hiccups, 52
High fever, 63
High pitched peristaltic sounds, 180
Hip pain, 59, 77-78, 150
Histamine, 13
Histologic study, 97
Historical review, 3-4
Horizontal method, 24
Hypertension, 45, 51, 62, 139, 148, 150
Hypertension insomnia, 45, 51
Hypnosis, 177, 179, 190
Hysteria, 59

I

Impotence, 55, 59, 68, 70-73, 148-149, 189
Improvement results, 188-191
Impulses, 121
Incense, 13-14
Incontinency, 68, 70, 98
Indigestion, 149
Infection, 24-25
Inflammatory joint, 101
Inguinal pain, 139
Inhibitory gates, 190
Insomnia, 45, 51, 59, 71, 84, 147-148
Intercostal neuralgia, 139
Intermittent needle motion, 32
Intestinal disease, 59, 148-149
Intestinal motility, 98-101, 176, 180-185
Intra-abdominal pain, 139
Intravital microscope, 124, 126
Intrinsic chemical substances, 13

K

Kidney disease, 59
Knee pain, 69, 73
Kocher clamping, 113

L

Large fibers, 121
Laryngeal spasm, 111
Lateral lower leg pain, 69
L-C neurometer, 124, 133, 190
Leg joint pain, 66, 69, 71, 76-77, 150
Leg paralysis, 66-71
Limpic lobe, 13
Line, 4
Lip tremor, 49
Liver disease, 58
Local anesthesia, 11, 138
Location, 105
Lower abdominal pain, 55, 81
Lower extremities, 67, 71
Lower leg paralysis, 71
Low hypogastrium, 55
Lumbosacral spine, 9, 186, 191

M

Malaria, 148
Mandibular joint pain, 46, 69
Manual stimulation, 106, 112
Massage, 33
Mastitis, 54
Mechanical energy, 9
Menstral pain, 150
Meridian lines, 3, 5-10, 12, 16, 18
  biliary meridian, 5, 8, 10, 18
  cardiac meridian, 5, 6, 10, 18
  colonic meridian, 5, 6, 10, 18
  endocrine meridian, 5, 6, 18
  gallbladder meridian, 5, 7, 10, 18
  gastric meridian, 5, 7, 10, 18
  hepatic meridian, 5, 8, 10, 18
  intestinal meridian, 5, 6, 10, 18
  pericardium meridian, 10
    conception vessel (cv) 42, 43
    governing vessel (gv) 42, 43
  pulmonary meridian, 5, 6, 10, 18
  renal meridian, 5, 9, 10, 18
  splenic meridian, 5, 8, 10, 18
  triple warmer meridian, 10
  urinary bladder meridian, 5, 9, 10, 18
  vascular meridian, 5, 6, 18
Meridian line theory, 16
Meridian points, 11-12, 16, 20, 40
Metabolic determinations, 127
Metalic ball, 16
Meteorism, 54, 55
Microcirculatory responses, 97, 126
Midvolar wrist, 142
Migraine, 46, 50, 62, 79
Mitochondria, 20
Moxa, 13-16
Mumps, 46
Muscle changes, 97-99
Musculoskeletal pain, 75-78
Mutism, 51-52, 61, 63
Myelinated fibers, 121
Myography, 6
Myopia, 46, 47, 88

N

Nair cream, 123
Nasal disease, 51
Nausea, 63
Neck pain, 61, 77, 147-148, 150, 186
Needle feeling, 32, 137
Needle feeling impulse, 91
Needle holder, 30-31
Needle insertion techniques, 24-32
Needle motions, 32-33
Needle sensation, 178
Needle shock, 90, 178, 188
Needles, 22-25, 92-93
Negative forces, 17
Nerve blocks, 13, 139
  brachial plexus, 141
  celiac plexus, 139, 148
  cervical, 140, 147
  common peroneal, 145
  common tibial, 172, 174
  deep peroneal, 145, 150

epidural, 139, 148
femoral, 143, 144, 150
infraorbital, 140, 147
mandibular, 147
maxillary, 140, 147
medial, 141, 142, 147
obturator, 143, 149
occipital, 147
paravertical, 138, 148
radial, 141, 147, 148
sacral, 138, 139, 149, 150
saphenous, 145, 150
sciatic, 144, 146, 150
somatic, 139, 148
suprascapular, 146
supraorbital, 140, 147
supratrochlear, 140, 147
sympathetic, 139, 148
ulnar, 141, 142, 147
neurometer, 5, 10, 20, 34, 41, 123, 133-134, 187, 190
Neuromuscular blockade, 176, 179
Neurophysiological data, 137, 162-163, 171-179
Neurosis, 54, 58-59, 147, 149
Nocturia, 73
Non-myelinated fibers, 121
Nose diseases, 51
Nystagmus, 45, 46

O

Objective, 187
Oblique, 24
Obstetrical problems, 71
Occipital headache, 71
Ohm's law, 103
One-hand method, 26
Optic nerve atrophy, 47, 87
Optic neuritis, 47
Optimal locations on needle points, 101-112
Oscilloscope, 103
Osteoarthritis, 130-138, 186, 191
Otorrhea, 49

P

Pain and numbness of fingers and finger joints, 63
Pain at fourth and fifth fingers, 60
Pain impulse, 21
Pain management, 121
Pain mechanisms, 12-14
Pain Study Center, Department of Surgery, Hahnemann Medical College & Hospital, 138
Pancreatic pain, 139
Pancreatitis, 58
Paralysis of extremities, 63
Paralysis of lower extremities, 66
Paralysis of upper arm, 64
Paralysis of upper extremities, 64
Paralytic ileus, 139
Paralyzing pressure sensation to glands penis or urethra, 55
Parameter, 187
Paravertebral block, 138
Paraviose, 20
Passing holes, 4, 127
Pathophysiology of acupuncture, 16
Patient positions, 34-39
Patoxysma, 109
Peak wave, 111
Peeping holes, 4, 127
Pendular movements, 183
Peptic ulcer, 58, 139
Peripheral vascular disease, 139
Peristaltic waves, 180
Perpendicular method, 24
Pharyngitis, 51, 52, 73, 81-82, 147
Phsiological data, 137
Plethysmographic measurement of the paw volumes, 101
Pleuritis, 56
Pneumonia, 56
Point locations, 40-42
Polygraph, 102
Polypeptides, 13
Positive forces, 17
Possible indications for acupuncture, 21-22
Post acupuncture massage, 33
Postoperative pain, 90, 189
Post vagotomy gastrointestinal atony, 128
Pre-acupuncture massage, 33
Premedication, 112
Preparation of needle, 37
Pruritus, 73
Psychosis, 54, 63
PTT, 132
Pulmonary emboli, 139
Pulse, 6
Pulse diagnosis, 17
Pulse interval, 129
Pushing hand, 29

R

Raynaud's disease, 139
Reactive electropermissible points, 20
Receptor, 13
Rectal diseases, 60
Rectangular current, 111
Regional anesthesia, 11, 138
Regional block vs. acupuncture, 138-150

Regulator, 121
Reilly phenomenon, 19
Renal diseases, 60
Renal stone, 139
Retching, 111
Retention method, 46, 49, 60
Retinal hemorrhage, 59
Resistor, 111
Respiration rate, 103
Rhinitis, 46, 61, 69, 87-88
Rhizotomy, 13
Ryodoketsu, 137
Ryodoraku theory, 12

S

Sacral block, 138
Scapulocostal syndrome, 145-146, 150
Sciatica, 59, 139
Sedative control of pain, 13
Segmental movements, 183
Selection of acupuncture points, 91-96
Selection of optimal animal needle locations, 112-122
Sensitive points, 42
Sensory evoked potential, 129
Sensory nerve, 11
Serotonin, 13
Shock, 63
Shoulder ache, 64
Shoulder joint pain, 64
Side effects, 90
Signal generator, 102, 104, 171
Sine wave, 171
Single blind study, 132
Single stick, 32
Sinking pulse, 17
Six hollow organs, 17
Six solid organs, 17
Skin disease, 62
Skin resistance, 111, 124
Sleep spindle, 176
SMA-12, 132
Social service, 167-168
Sparrow pecking, 32, 188
Special flow system, 17
Spinal cord, 20
Sprains, 52, 77-78
Square wave, 171
Stilmulation therapy, 4, 13, 14
Strabismus, 47
Stressor, 139
Stress theory (Hans Selye), 19
Substantia gelatinosa, 21, 121
Sympathetic nerve, 11
Sympathetic nervous system, 127
Symptoms complex, 17
Syncope, 49, 58, 59, 65

T

Tachycardia, 58
Tapping method, 25
Te-chi's phenomenon, 178
Techniques of needle insertion, 24
Thalamotomy, 13
Thalamus, 121, 122, 190
Theories, 16
Thigh pain, 65
Throat pain, 73
Tic Douloureaux, 73
Tinnitis, 47, 49, 60, 63
Tonsilitis, 60-62, 81-82, 147
Toothache, 147
Topical hypothermia, 13
Tractotomy, 13
Tranquilizers, 13
Transmittor cell, 121
Treatment methods, 12
Tremor of lips, 49
Trigeminal neuralgia, 51
Truncal vagotomy, 127
Twirling (free-hand) method, 26, 29-32

U

Ulnar volar wrist, 142
Ultropak intravital microscope, 125
Unconsciousness, 73, 85
Upper abdominal pain, 63
Upper arm pain, 64
Upper arm paralysis, 64
Uterine proplapse, 56
Urethal pain, 68, 70
URI 54
Uric acid, 186
Urinalysis, 186
Urinary disorders, 59
Urinary retention, 66

V

Vibration, 32
Viscerocutaneous autonomic reflex, 20
Voltage, 103
Vomiting, 52, 54, 63, 83

W

Water needle, 94
Wave forms, 105
Wrist joint pain, 62, 148